"When KJ Landis was ready to make a personal change happen in her diet and lifestyle, she turned to self-experimenting using the HCG protocol with spectacular results.Through her experience of dramatic fat loss and health change, KJ realized that it is possible to become your own *Superior Self* with the right information about nutrition and fitness, customized to your specific metabolic needs. *Superior Self* is your rallying cry to do something NOW about your health, so that your future will be filled with promise for a better tomorrow. KJ delivers the cold hard truth about sugar, fat, calories, and more, all shared in love and empathy from someone who knows from whence she speaks."

~Jimmy Moore, Livin' La Vida Low-Carb blog and podcast
Author of *Cholesterol Clarity* (2013 –Victory
Belt Publishing) and
Keto Clarity (2014 - Victory Belt Publishing)

"KJ Landis shows us that restoring health is possible. If you're ready to discover your *Superior Self*, this is your guide to creating a happy and healthy mind, body, and spirit."

~Joe and Heather Juliani, Founders of Phase4Life
Authors of *Phase 4 Life: Life's a Journey, Not a Diet* (2014)

"In my experience as a health professional, I have seen firsthand that much of emotional and mental health can be controlled through healthy eating. As more people discover the connection between the food that they eat and their mental health, *Superior Self* will prove to be invaluable.

If you are reading this, consider yourself one of the lucky ones who is nutritionally conscious and well on your way superior health.

This book provides both men and women with a practical guide for realizing what they are eating, how much they are eating, and what foods work best while choosing superior health."

~Selena Le Blanc, M.A; MFTi
Parenting Skills Consultant Providing Supportive
Services to the Developmentally Delayed Population
Author of *Mindfulness Based Stress Reduction
Group for Adolescent Mothers* (2011)

"Excessive fat in our bodies not only poses as a health risk leading to many ailments, but also lowers our self esteem in that we are not beautiful or handsome enough. It can make us feel pessimistic towards life. KJ Landis shows us through her writing that she cares about the people who don't consider themselves "cool."

The information here has greatly helped my patients who have chronic diseases predisposed by excessive fat in their bodies coupled with inactivity. Be blessed and encouraged as you read *Superior Self.*"

~Dr. Abel O. Apima, MBChB, General Practitioner
In-Charge, Chronic Diseases at Saifee Foundation
Medical Centre, Mombasa, Kenya.

SUPERIOR
SELF

Reaching Superior Health
For A Superior Self

KJ LANDIS, BS

BALBOA
PRESS

A DIVISION OF HAY HOUSE

Balboa Press books may be ordered through booksellers or by contacting:

Balboa Press
A Division of Hay House
1663 Liberty Drive
Bloomington, IN 47403
www.balboapress.com
1 (877) 407-4847

Because of the dynamic nature of the Internet, any web addresses or links contained in this book may have changed since publication and may no longer be valid. The views expressed in this work are solely those of the author and do not necessarily reflect the views of the publisher, and the publisher hereby disclaims any responsibility for them.

The author of this book does not dispense medical advice or prescribe the use of any technique as a form of treatment for physical, emotional, or medical problems without the advice of a physician, either directly or indirectly. The intent of the author is only to offer information of a general nature to help you in your quest for emotional and spiritual well-being. In the event you use any of the information in this book for yourself, which is your constitutional right, the author and the publisher assume no responsibility for your actions.

Any people depicted in stock imagery provided by Thinkstock are models, and such images are being used for illustrative purposes only. Certain stock imagery © Thinkstock.

Printed in the United States of America.

ISBN: 978-1-4525-2135-0 (sc)
ISBN: 978-1-4525-2137-4 (hc)
ISBN: 978-1-4525-2136-7 (e)

Library of Congress Control Number: 2014915751

Balboa Press rev. date: 09/22/2014

TO MY LOVES

Torino, Golden, and Sage

"There is nothing noble in being superior to your fellow man; true nobility is being superior to your former self."

~Ernest Hemingway

CONTENTS

FOREWORD

*S*uperior *Self* is the perfect title for KJ Landis' first book. Life is not about achieving perfection, but it is about listening to your higher calling, finding the superior self within each and every one of us.

Superior Self addresses the emotional aspects of eating and weight loss extremely well. It goes hand-in-hand with our HCG Body for Life philosophy: permanent results without permanent dieting. What this book provides are some very powerful tips and concrete suggestions for figuring out what's really going on inside of us when we overeat, what to do about it, and then lays out a real game plan for long-term fat loss and wellness.

Considered by many to be one of the foremost HCG protocol experts in the country, KJ Landis is by far my most successful coaching client. She has not only embraced our lifestyle, but has taken it to a whole new level of healthy living. The author does this by sharing her personal transformation, knowledge, and expertise with people around the world.

Superior Self has a unique and special way of making complex issues simple by breaking things down into easy to understand concepts. Anyone who is looking to achieve long-term fat loss and maintenance can easily reach his or her desired goal by following the step-by-step roadmap for success laid out here.

Unlike many health and fitness books, *Superior Self* gives readers everyday tools to overcome their challenges with their body images. *Superior Self: Reaching Superior Health for a Superior Self* will make you think deeply about the true life goals that can be chased after once the health and fat loss struggles are over. The time is now. You are here. *Superior Self* is your ally in breaking through your limited beliefs, and in loving yourselves enough to finally reveal your *own* superior self.

Colin F. Watson ~
Author of *How to Feel Good Naked in 26 Days* and Creator of HCG Body for Life

PREFACE

*T*his is not a diet book. I used myself as a weight and fat loss experiment. When I had results that were favorable, my friends and family asked what I was doing to achieve optimal health and wellness. This book is the long answer to their questions.

Being a woman, my weight always had close emotional bonds to the rest of me. Why do we give so much power to some digits on a mechanical device that basically measures our gravitational pull upon the earth? I am not my weight, but my whole day could be affected one way or the other on the emotional pendulum, just after weighing myself. I know that I am not alone. Perhaps you were singing in the car on the way to work when the digits pleased you. Perhaps you slammed the front door and cursed every red light when the digits did not please you.

Some anecdotal evidence is shared here, as well as my learning from research by reading books, papers, articles, blogs, lectures, and listening to many podcasts. The podcasts were talks and interviews with scientists, doctors, professors, researchers, cutting edge fitness and health professionals. My book is based on observational studies, not clinical trials. I am not a doctor, this is not medical advice, and I suggest you consult your health practitioner before embarking upon any new protocol of wellness. This is for informational use only and the material here is not intended to diagnose or treat any medical condition. I encourage a healthy and open new kind of dialogue between patient and practitioner.

Even if you are a health, medical, or fitness professional, you can definitely gain benefit from the information within this book. Personal health success stories that are long term and emotionally uplifting can go a long way in inspiring and motivating others.

The main goal I have for you in reading this book is to reach for your superior self. I believe the way to live, honoring our most authentic mind, body, and spirit, is to reach for superior health, thus leading to attainment of one's superior self. Great health, and eating in a way that nourishes our bodies to optimum levels can make us perform better in every area of our lives.

We are naturally focused on food from the moment we are born. We root for our mothers' nipples minutes after entering the world. We live or die based upon first whether we eat or starve. It makes sense then, that every day we have urges to eat in order to stay alive. The importance of what we put into our bodies is key to how the rest of our existence fares. Eat well, live well. Eat junk, and our capacity to learn, to remember, and to move physically is impaired, eventually. This journey of life through food can be overwhelmingly positive or negative. It is an individual and unique journey. Bon voyage!

ACKNOWLEDGEMENTS

I want to thank my family, friends, and tribe of followers out there on the World Wide Web. You had a trust and faith in me that are unparalleled in many other areas of my life. The support and suggestions have made me a better writer, a better listener, and a better human being.

Thank you to my husband and children, who gave me the encouragement and patience when needed. You were committed to me and my dreams from the very beginning.

Thank you to my mentor, coach, and friend Colin F. Watson for answering my questions and calling me back! You truly know how to pay it forward. Thank you to Jayne Johnson Watson because she is the foundation that supports and spurs Colin forward.

Thank you to the truth tellers of the world. We are so bombarded with information these days that it is difficult to sift the truth from the snake oil.

And finally, thank you to the farmers and food producers of the world who are creating chemical-free, real, whole food options for the world to eat in a sustainable manner.

MY STORY

On my 46th birthday, I ran my 14th marathon. Then I rewarded myself with cake, martinis, clams, cheese, crackers, and fruit. At 183 pounds, I was proportionate in my body parts and looked good for my height of 5 feet 10 inches.

But...I wasn't happy with my weight or size. As a former fashion model, now working as a server for about fifteen years, I had gained close to five pounds a year and had bore two children.

So, as a kind of mid-life crisis gift to myself, I decided to have a liposuction. I paid the down payment to the doctor and settled on a date. Afterwards, I told my husband. He heatedly stated that I would just "blow up" again if I didn't change my eating habits. He thought it was a waste of my money, and a crutch to avoid the real problem: my eating choices when at work and when he wasn't around. After deep self reflection, I admitted to myself that he was right.

I researched other weight loss options that the plastic surgeon offered on her website, and HCG was named there. It intrigued me. I had never heard of HCG before. I then read the original Dr. Simeons protocol from 1954 in its entirety on line. I became fully aware of the history of the HCG hormone and its use in fat loss. I then researched everything I could about it on the internet and the name Colin F. Watson kept popping up. His free podcasts, website, advice, blogs, and even phone number were available! So, I listened to his podcasts called HCG Body for Life, in chronological order from the very first one back in 2010. After weeks of listening, learning and absorbing as much of the information as I could, I embarked upon the HCG protocol.

Before I took the HCG injections (which I received from my local plastic surgeon), I cleansed my body for three weeks. I ate very clean, with no processed foods at all, no meats or dairy, no fats, grains, or sugars. I drank a gallon of water daily. At the end of the cleanse I began the HCG shots and program. I lost 50 pounds in 60 days! My second month's worth of HCG I purchased from HCG Body for Life. I called Colin F. Watson and e-mailed him with questions during my journey. He rapidly answered my questions without charging me. He even called me back! He didn't mind that I bought the first batch of HCG from someone else. His passion and his goals are to cure obesity and the chronic conditions caused by obesity. Colin asked of me only one thing: pay it forward.

So here we are. I am more than two years from my desperate cry for help. I have successfully maintained the fat and weight loss. I continue to live grain free and sugar free ninety percent of the time. I do have planned treats that are regret free. I have added Bikram hot yoga to my daily workout routine. I still drink a gallon of water a day, sometimes more.

Colin F. Watson invited me to be a guest on his radio show numerous times to share my discoveries, tips, and tricks that have kept me from relapsing into old habits. I even talked about underground natural therapies for cancer and chronic illnesses. I continue to study and read cutting edge nutrition and health science materials. The public library has become a close friend. I listen to lectures and podcasts, mostly staying within the Paleo eating template of consuming real whole foods.

Since my weight loss was so great and rapid, my friends and family inquired about the protocol I was following. I began coaching people to fulfill their own health and wellness goals based on the things I have learned and experimented with. Some followed the HCG Body for Life protocol. Some followed the original Simeons protocol. Some gave up grains and sugar. Some just began moving more, and drank a gallon of water a day. All of them gifted me with their trust, and I do not take that lightly. People generally don't know who to trust because there are so many gimmicky diets out there in the supermarkets, pharmacies, and on the internet. The diets presented in the general media ads are short term. When we turn our food world completely around long term, we embrace a lifestyle change instead of a diet. It has been called a therapeutic lifestyle change, or TLC! We are giving ourselves tender loving care.

One purpose of this book is to learn how to sustain your health goals long term, so you can eat in a way where you never have to worry about weight gain again. I want to impress upon you the variety of healthy eating protocols available these days. The variety of eating protocols healing to the body somehow works as well in assisting in fat loss. I also wish for you to incorporate fun in your day, in some way, and to gain spiritual truths that resonate with you. I want you to pay it forward in your own unique way.

Colin encouraged me to write a blog about my experiences with the weight loss and beyond. This was important to him because I shared spiritual insights that occurred simultaneously while on the weight loss journey. I spoke with his radio audience about the spiritual side of my journey numerous times. When I stopped filling myself with food and stifling my inner voice, there became a space open inside of me, ready and willing to listen to my inner voice and the voice of divine inspiration. I received messages daily from God.

My son recently taught me how to use Facebook as a platform to post blogs on my very first fan page. I call it Superior Self with KJ Landis. The name came to me while jogging at the beach. I was praying for guidance from above. Most of my divine interventions and inspirations hit me when I am running. Now I write blogs and list tips that have helped me along my way. I share photos with the world of meals and recipes I create. My children film me weekly, sharing my two minute nutritional nuggets of information that

I post on SuperiorSelf on YouTube. I answer coaching questions and encourage other humans to reach for *their* superior health in order to discover *their* superior self. I believe we all have the capacity to know something, do something, and be something...our most authentic selves.

Think of this book as a fun and informational tool box that you can turn to when you doubt yourself. I dream for you what I achieved through hard work and dedication. This tool box contains a brief description of the original prescription HCG protocol, the HCG Body for Life protocol, and my tips and tricks that will assist in the phases of the protocol. The full Simeons protocol is available freely on line as well as the HCG Body for Life protocol in its entirety. I will share what I eat now and what good and bad foods do to the body. I will cover underground wellness therapies for chronic conditions and the ancestral way of eating for longevity and optimum health.

Please know that I am not going to change your life. *You* are going to change your life. The human spirit thrives upon challenges. We seek them out in many ways, all of the time. When we meet these challenges head on and step into uncharted territory, our growth is exponential. Every small step is a step in your favorable direction. Health and wellness problems can keep us stuck in other facets of our lives. When we figure out how to get unstuck in this area, we can awaken the value of our lives to the utmost degree. Every corner of our lives will begin to open up.

I named this book and the blog *Superior Self* because my wellness journey sent me on a quest to go further in my education of what exactly nutrient dense, real food is, what are smart exercise habits, and what are some disease prevention protocols. This is not just another diet book. It is not a diet book at all. It is a life lesson in nourishment sustainability with happy side effects. I no longer struggle to maintain my sanity while staying healthy. When we are healthy at the very smallest cellular level, things begin to fall into their rightful place. I strive to provide you with solid information and consistency throughout the book. Many suggestions given here I have experimented with on myself, on my coaching clients, family, and friends. Welcome to *Superior Self.* You can...you can...you can...

Chapter One

THE MIND
VS
THE BODY

*L*osing weight is simple, right? Eat certain foods, stay away from other particular foods, and remember to exercise a lot. The combination of these activities produces weight loss. It is pretty easy in the math too. Take in fewer calories that you put out, and the result is the body of your dreams...Bogus, bogus, bogus.

When I did the government and medically recommended methods of weight loss, I did lose weight for a little while. Then a little while later, I gained the weight back. Because of my talent in following the rules, so many of my experiences resulted in disappointment in myself and lower self esteem. I did not pig out to gain the weight back. I just ate "normally" again. I never stopped going to the gym or running. In fact, I was a certified spinning instructor and completed fourteen marathons during the years that I steadily gained weight. I even ate "healthy whole grains" and "low fat, heart healthy" products.

So, what was it? What was my downfall over and over again? Besides being fooled by the American Dietary Association, the American Medical Association, the Food and Drug Administration, and mainstream media, it was my own mind. I had to change my mind in order to consistently change my habits. I couldn't finish a three hour kick-ass workout and hit the Chinese food buffet anymore. I had to hit a deep, dark hurting spot, that wall in my mind that says, "I am done with this roller coaster ride. I don't want to exercise more and more hours a day year in and year out and still gain a few pounds and inches each and every year. I am desperate. DONE."

That was my turning point. Next came my big WHY. Why did I decide to seek a permanent change once and for all? Basically, I wanted to be more of *me*, my most authentic, loving, giving, un-self-conscious self. In order to do that, I had to shift my eating paradigm and seek out a different protocol for life. If I could change the psychology, I could change the body.

Ask yourself, *why?* Why this time? Why this time in this particular period of your life? Who do you want to be healthy, happy, and fit for? What other life goals will you go after when you achieve your superior health? Do you desire to reach your superior self? This challenge is a journey for the mind, body, and spirit. It is a task well worth attending to because you are ready now. You are a shining, sparkling, invaluable being, worthy of every goodness and blessing. You are worth it! I truly believe that, or I would not have begun coaching for free, blogging, and sharing my story of discoveries.

Put your attention on your intention. What is your intention? I intend to have superior health and happiness. Why? I intend to have superior health and happiness because I desire to live long and be supple in my movements. That robust longevity will enable me to be of service to others and to fully enjoy my family, friends, and those whom I serve.

Now, to fully pay attention to that, I had to do something about my weight. That was when I was opened up enough in my soul spot, my vulnerability, to acknowledge and accept the HCG Body for Life protocol into my personal space. I was ready to fully trust the process. Perhaps you are ready for a program of eating and wellness that will serve your higher purpose. It does not have to be the same one I was committed to, but it must resonate with your whole being.

What we think over and over again becomes what we believe. Our thoughts become our beliefs, and then our whole being gets the message by aligning within that belief system. Then our actions support that belief system. Why do we seem shocked when we get results based upon that activity? We think it's a miracle, but it is our own personal answer based upon a spark of new information or insight. Kind of like, "wash, rinse, repeat, wash, rinse, repeat." Sooner or later we will believe the clothes (or hair) will be clean. Your intention may not be fat loss or a smaller clothes size. Your intention may be to gain energy, lose aches and pains, or sleep through the night. Whatever the goal, put your attention on your intention.

The HCG falling into my sphere, when I had never come across the word before, was the divine spark. Then I went beyond the surface of the HCG protocol and it became a journey that was something else entirely. I read, listened to, and watched everything I could get my hands on in ancient and new alternative methods of eating for health, fat loss, optimum nutrition, and natural healing of all kinds of conditions. The fire inside of me is still stoked daily by new questions that pop into my head. Then, I'm off and running to seek out the answers for those whose lives I touch as well as for myself.

Hide-and-seek...We played this game for years as children. When we found our friends hiding, we were happy to see them. Be happy to find your true self, hiding in the corners, under things, behind things, in the closet, under the bed, under the covers. When you discover the authentic *you*, you will be greeted by a hidden best friend, who was waiting patiently, ready and willing to play some more, laugh some more, and love some more. So what are you waiting for? Whether it is the body of your dreams, the love of your dreams, the career of your dreams, or to be your personal best, know that others are there to play with you, uphold you, and support you to your highest version of yourself.

We can self-talk into limitations or into limitless possibilities. Sometimes when attempting something for the first time (or the umpteenth time), we say that we *can't*. Really what this means is that we *won't*. We do not want to do X, Y, or Z. Not now, not yet. Realize that this is an imaginary limitation. The imagination is a great source of explosive creativity and yeses. The imagination is also a great source of negative stories that feed self doubt. I am asking you to reverse the conversation you have with yourself that keeps you in less than optimum health and vitality. As you believe in yourself a little bit more each and every day, the yeses will outnumber the noes, and perhaps at the end of your time here on Earth, you will be completely satisfied and blissful on the way out.

I do not want more and more and more things at the end of my life. Rather, I want more and more and more of *me* at the end of my life. Old habits are comfortable and non confrontational, yet they yield old results. New habits are uncomfortable and may create tension in your internal and external worlds, but they yield new results. Place the imaginary limitations into the incinerator, ditch the old habits, and embrace the positive you, the person you know that is inside of you, patiently waiting for this moment.

How do we change the internal language that we have had for so long? The feeling in our heart that we *can't*, we aren't good enough, etc. can be altered with conscious and repeated effort. If you attempt this admirable feat a little at a time, the internal dialogue will change permanently. If you were at a restaurant and the food you ordered came out completely wrong, you probably would send it back. You would patiently (or impatiently) wait for the correct order. I suggest doing that with the negative internal conversation. Send it back to the kitchen (brain) to be made right. Tell yourself that it is unacceptable in this presentation.

When I was overweight, rarely did strangers on the city streets give me attention. I felt comfortable in my own skin. I felt attractive, liked, and trusted within my circle of family and friends. Being overweight made me invisible in a way that was perfectly okay with me for a long time. After all, I was married for close to two decades and had two children. Being just another middle aged, frumpily shaped woman was acceptable to me. When I lost the weight and fat, my youthful modeling shape reemerged. All of a sudden, I was getting whistled at, received cat calls, and more attention from both men and women I didn't know at all. This created a new kind of tension and anxiety within me. I had not had this sort of public attention in years, and it was uncomfortable at first. Even though I was proud of my weight loss, I had not anticipated the extra energy being thrown at me freely.

Perhaps we feel safe being at a size or shape that makes us invisible in a crowd. It takes a lot of mental effort to be willing to shed that layer of safety along with the layers of fat and weight loss.

The mind and body do not have to be at constant odds with each other. Do we really have to have the mind versus the body? It is our heart that can be the mediator between the two. I believe we can utilize the heart and ask it to massage both the mind and the body into a cooperative relationship. The heart perseveres with grace, strength, and tenacity. Sit quietly with yourself a few minutes each day. Pray for your heart to reach the rest of you.

Two things to consider when we talk about the mind versus the body are willpower and won't power. Our mind is strong and flexible. It *will* work with us to meet our goals. It *won't*, however, change our basic genetic makeup. An apple is not a pear is not a stick of gum. A person who is pear-shaped will not become apple-shaped or stick-shaped no matter how hard he or she works at it. We can improve upon the basic framework that our genes gave us, but we cannot completely change everything. We are predisposed to a particular body type. We must work within that parameter, and be aware of it so that we do not feel like a failure.

Getting your mind right and ready for your superior self will allow your life goals to happen naturally in a flow so that you may redeem all of the benefits and qualities of the body your spirit is living in. Confidence, self esteem, greater health, ease of movement in mind, body, and spirit *is attainable*, my friends. I am living proof. Now it is your turn. I offer you your superior self.

Chapter Two

THE TRUTH

*W*hen we are overweight, some of us believe that the reason we are fat is because we didn't work hard enough, or that we didn't have enough willpower to not eat junk food and treats. That, simply stated, is a lie. We are not weaker than thin and fit people. Populations around the world have been extremely disciplined and successful at losing pounds in the short term, repeatedly. We are not overweight because of gluttony and sloth. We are overweight because of our physiology naturally reacting to the low fat, whole grain, artificially sweetened foods that we consume when we follow the mainstream media and medical community's recommendations. It has been this dogmatic approach for so many decades that has brought us to this epidemic situation of obesity in our modern society.

If we are expending more and more energy, and not taking in equal energy, our brain sends signals to the body to eat, eat, eat. Eventually we receive the message. We are usually ravished by this point, and we pounce upon insane things, where we would have probably chosen better foods had we not been so deprived. We may relieve ourselves of the guilt and self hatred caused by breaking our deprivation. We are not meant to starve for years, months, weeks, or even days on end.

Our body wants to remain in balance. It is self regulating of all of its systems. This internal stability of our body systems is called homeostasis. Our willpower is limited and sooner or later our brain signals surpass the willpower and our body instructs us to eat. So we eat. What we choose to eat after suffering the imbalance is the key to why our bodies are metabolically broken. After a diet of struggle and not eating enough nutrients to feed our cells, we usually turn to a highly processed grain product, coupled with refined sugars or toxic fats or a combination of these three things. This cycle, when used habitually, can cause adrenal fatigue, inflammation, as well as a myriad of illnesses and conditions, including weight gain.

The standard American diet has duped us, unfortunately. The abbreviation for it is SAD, and it is very sad indeed! Food that is made from highly processed, non-nutritive substances has a great chance of making us fat, sick, ugly, and old... eventually. These non-foods, let's call them edible-food-wannabes, are filling us up but not fulfilling our essential nutritional needs. Therefore we get signals from our brain very soon after ingesting them that we are still hungry. So we eat again. The cycle continues. I think of this cycle similar to a life of one night stands versus a long and satisfying relationship. Do we want instant gratification or overall lasting health?

Obesity is not the entire problem. A broken metabolism is the problem, and obesity is a side effect of that. Most health care costs in the USA result from diseases and conditions caused by a broken metabolism. One does not necessarily have to be fat to suffer from a metabolic disorder. Many of us know people who are "skinny-fat." They may be thin as a rail but are taking high cholesterol medications, have type 2 diabetes, high blood pressure, arthritis, gout, memory loss, etc. Immunity to any disease begins in the gut. What we take into our bodies is of the utmost importance.

The calories in, calories out model of health and vitality serve us no more. It does, however, serve the mainstream farmers, the food manufacturing industry, the FDA, the advertisers, mainstream media, and Wall Street. Anybody hear of 100 calorie packs? Why haven't those 100 calorie packs kept us free from obesity? Some *expert* thought they were a great idea.

If I drank only a can of cola and ate an apple daily, in a few days I would lose weight. It has roughly 300 calories, less than my body needed to maintain my weight. Besides that, I would feel hungry, fatigued, and grumpy. On the inside, however, my organs and hormones would not be working very well. The hormones that process and regulate my energy, fat, and appetite would be out of whack. The body's imbalances don't happen after one fast food meal. These things take time and the body can really take a lot of abuse before things break down.

In my own case, I was blindly setting up my imbalances from a very young age. I began life as a normal weight child. Then from about age five to twelve I steadily became larger and larger, slower and slower. My family fed me well, according to the four food groups that were the guidelines of my youth. My parents came from Russian and Eastern European backgrounds, where meat and potatoes, stews, stuffings, breads, pastries, and cakes were daily occurrences.

The 1970s modern conveniences of canned, packaged, and frozen goods assisted my mother greatly in preparing meals for a family of seven. The price points of these convenient products added to their appeal. Margarine and lard type shortening products, as well as new, cheaper, and "healthier" vegetable oils added to my personal demise. Instant cold and hot cereals, cake mixes, instant rice, mashed potatoes, and of course soda pop were all around me. I was happy to be a part of the new age. I belonged to the clean plate club too. My mother was so proud of her good eater!

Little did I know that by age 12 those daily habits would literally age me. Remember that I mentioned earlier that these substances would make us fat, sick, ugly, and old? Well, it eventually broke my metabolism. I was 12 years old, five feet two inches tall, and weighed 173 pounds.

My parents took me to my yearly checkup, where we all received a verbal slap on the wrist from the pediatrician, and I was sent directly to the endocrinologist and dietician. There, I learned that I would be at least five feet eight inches tall when I was done growing. I also learned that I had the insides of an obese, ill, 48 year old person, with cholesterol and triglycerides running so high that the ink ran off of the ink graph charts. The endocrinologist scared my family straight. He stated that if I kept up my bad eating habits, I was playing fire with heart disease and heart attack risk. He also said that my knees probably would begin to ache if I gained more weight because my legs were skinny compared to the rest of me and they may not be able to support my body.

For the next two years solid I kept a food diary. I ate no more than 1200 calories a day, and chose fruits and vegetables over everything else. I exercised as a means of weight loss, not for play's sake. I would not permit myself to go to sleep until I completed 200 sit-ups. I met monthly with my pediatric dietician for weigh-ins and intake of my food journal. During those two years I lost 40 pounds and grew eight inches. The pediatric staff declared me one of their most successful outcomes. My hard work and discipline paid off. Yet nobody at the clinic shared with me that the composition and the quality of the calories were just as important, if not more important than the number of calories. No one told me how vital water intake was to weight loss and overall health either.

I was still metabolically broken, but now it was working in the opposite direction. By age 14, I was five feet ten inches tall and 133 pounds. From ages 14 to 16, I tested my personal limits. I went weeks of liquid only diets, fruit only diets, the grapefruit diet, the cabbage soup diet, the rotation diet, and whatever else was the fad of the moment. My metabolism was at last on rapid fire, and I went down to my lowest weight of 102 pounds. I was ecstatic! Some nights, I would eat up to eight almond croissants, heated with lots of butter and preserves. The next day I would weigh myself. To my delight, I didn't gain weight and sometimes I would even lose a few pounds. Talk about lucky (!), or so I thought. The road to disaster is a winding one and fraught with potholes. Over the years I was methodically, yet unknowingly wrecking my metabolism.

What does that mean exactly? What is metabolism? Metabolism is the breaking down of molecules to get energy and use it for our lives. Nutrition is the key to metabolism. We eat, and the nutrients in our food are broken down into smaller and smaller particles, fed to our cells, and then we use these jazzed up cells as energy to create our movements, utilize our muscles, give us brain power, etc. To understand our metabolism better and how it can get broken, we need to look at metabolism regulating hormones.

Leptin is a hormone found in our fat cells. It is released from the fat cell, sends messages to the brain, and tells the hypothalamus gland in the brain that we are full, satisfied, and we have energy to do the work our body requires of us. If leptin is not released from the fat cells, or if the hypothalamus gland doesn't receive the information properly, we are still hungry.

Insulin is another hormone that works directly with leptin. It tells the fat cells to store energy that is coming in from our food, while also at the same time, tells the brain to stop the hunger. In properly working metabolisms, when we eat well, we get fidgety and active afterwards. If the signals get mixed up, we don't get the information, and the body keeps feeling hungry. We then feel lethargic, kind of like a couch potato because we are still hungry. Our bodies think we should not move that much when we are hungry, in order not to starve. We save our energy. If we starve ourselves with drastic dieting and lower quality calorie habits, our body and brain get the message to be a couch potato.

This is called insulin resistance. This is when our body's metabolism, or energy output, is reduced. In fact, the data shows that the same effort in physical activities will burn less calories (less energy output) if we aren't eating enough good quality food. This especially is affected if we aren't eating nutrient dense, good-fat containing, and satisfying foods. Refined sugars, processed carbohydrates, and junk foods all fall into that category of deregulating the body's system of balance, or homeostasis.

Imagine your food choices in this way: You bought tickets on the internet from a scalper for a musical concert. You were assured that they were front row seats, but when you arrived at the venue, the seats were the cheap seats. They were way up high, and far from the stage. I don't want you to stay in the cheap seats. You deserve better. Refined carbohydrates and sugar are the cheap seats. High quality proteins, vegetables, and fruits are like front row tickets with a VIP back stage pass to the concert. I want you to realize that *you* are the star of your very own show. You are the greatest experiment of your beautiful life.

Our belief system of what is good to eat has been skewed by the media bombardment every time we turn on our radios, televisions, computers, and smart phones. Add to that the food pyramid and the food plate funded by the agriculture and food manufacturing industries. It is no wonder we are all confused.

In fact, processed foods are designed by the manufacturers to be addictive. The high-sugar, low-fiber, packaged convenience foods stimulate serotonin and endorphin responses in the brain. These are pleasure hormones, and immediately after eating processed foods, we get us these hard wired pleasure responses. It is not our fault when we get a smile on our faces and enter into a food coma after desserts and chocolates.

The connection between sweets and the pleasure response begins with the newborn's natural reaction to mother's milk, which is extremely sweet. It is part of our human survival techniques. The packaged food industry is well aware of this. Processed foods are specifically engineered to keep us malnourished, so that we are not nutritionally satisfied. We then crave more, buy more, and eat more. They are also created to be bland in flavor so we can mindlessly munch, munch, and munch.

Furthermore, sugary and refined foods have been linked to feeding cancer and Alzheimer's disease. The wrong kinds of fats and oils combined with sugars usually are found in foods with preservatives too. Preservatives are things added to foods to make them last longer on the supermarket shelves. They did not come from nature. Preservatives are meant to preserve, to last, to sustain, and to hold on to something. So, please do not be surprised that in our bodies that *something* being preserved is fat. The only thing that should have a long shelf life is me! I want a long, healthy, and vibrant life span while on earth.

Remember though, even with all the finger pointing about how we have been fooled with the healthy, whole grain, fat free, sugar free foods out there, we ultimately have been the consumers financially supporting these companies. We do need to have a clearer understanding of our food sources and their sustainability in order to sustain our most healthy desires. Knowledge is power. Manufacturers do not tell us how many months or years their edible-food-wannabes have been on warehouse shelves before heading over to the local grocery stores. The big companies are not sharing the names of the chemical fertilizers used on their ingredients that are listed in the nutritional facts label.

Even fresh fruits and vegetables are not currently farmed in the way they were a hundred years ago. The commercially farmed produce does not meet our true nutrient needs. Nowadays, produce is farmed specifically to increase sugar and therefore calorie content. That continues the spike in insulin and the cravings afterward.

We need tools to provoke these feel good hormones without the refined carbohydrates and sugar. Eat crap, and we will look and feel crappy. Eat clean and pretty, and we will become clean and pretty. When my food and my fitness are in alignment, I feel fabulous every day, from the inside out. It is just a new choice coupled with desire, determination, and dedication that can lead us toward the path of optimum health and wellness. Love yourself into a better existence.

Earlier in this book I shared that I was a professional model for years. Even during the time that I was modeling, I played dangerously with my nutrition intake, unintentionally of course. A typical day began with coffee, cream, sugar, and a few packages of single serve preserves. I'd follow this with an exercise regime that included running, biking, weight training, and calisthenics. By lunch time I was starving but usually had to go on appointments to see potential clients. There was no time to sit down and properly nourish myself or to be present with my food in a mindful way. My routine had me regularly eating apples and popcorn purchased at a corner store along the way. In the evenings I would finally prepare a balanced meal of protein and vegetables, but because I was so "good" during the day, I would allow myself copious amounts of bread and butter, plus a dessert.

Even when I stopped modeling I still exercised and taught fitness classes part time. I ran marathons for years and in the back of my mind it was a means to reward myself with the notion that I could eat whatever I wanted because I was training so hard and for so long. How does one train for and run multiple marathons, and still gain 50 pounds over those same years? Something was out of whack, and that something was my metabolism, broken by years of incorrect food choices.

In the next part of this book I will tell you what I know about the HCG diet, the Paleolithic way of eating, a simple elimination protocol, facts about sugar, soy, coconut oil, and expose several alternative therapies for treating cancer and chronic degenerative diseases. Finally, I will gift you with tips and tricks that I have discovered and used in everyday life, during and after my weight loss journey. There are spiritual nuggets of wisdom I gained along my path. My a-ha moments have spurred me towards maintaining superior health. Ultimately, I feel completely at home inside of my superior self. Let's go!

Chapter Three

THE HCG PROTOCOL

When I embarked upon the HCG diet, I lost 50 pounds in 60 days! My life has not been the same since.

So, what is HCG and how does it work in weight and fat loss?

HCG is human chorionic gonadotropin. It is a hormone that is produced in larger quantities in pregnant women's placenta cells. When pregnant, women have HCG present in their blood tests and that is how they find out they are pregnant. HCG also aids in the testicle development in boys.

If women are malnourished or starving during pregnancy, the HCG helps the body utilize abnormal body fat to be as energy in order to feed the fetus in the uterus. This is the *extra* body fat I am referring to, not the fat that is surrounding our organs. Dr. A. T. W. Simeons discovered this in his research in the 1940s and 1950s in India. When HCG was administered by him to overweight teenage boys who had not yet had their gonads drop into their testicle sac, the surprising result was not only successful puberty progress, but also weight and fat loss. Dr. Simeons then took this hormone and injected it into obese men and non-pregnant, overweight women. He coupled the daily injections with a very specific low calorie, low fat eating plan. The outcome of this research was that the patients lost dramatic amounts of weight with retention of most of the muscle mass. He practiced this protocol for years in Rome, Italy in his very own obesity clinic.

The full book, which he published in 1954 for other medical professionals' use is called *POUNDS AND INCHES: A NEW APPROACH TO OBESITY.* It is widely available to read for free on the internet. Here is my summary of the original protocol's four phases.

SIMEONS' HCG PROTOCOL OVERVIEW

PHASE 1: The Gorging Phase

Upon awakening, use the restroom and weigh yourself to the tenth of a pound. Weigh yourself in the nude in a spot that will yield consistent results on the scale. Inject the HCG, prescribed by your doctor, into your fatty tissue. The original amount to inject was 125 international units. Proceed immediately to eat as much fatty, fried, sugary, rich foods as you can, all day long, until you retire at night. Fill up with anything that you think that you will miss during the very low calorie phase. Inject again the second morning, and indulge again, more than you think you can. You should be completely full and very uncomfortable at the end of these two days. You want the HCG to identify where the fat stores are, so it chases the fat filled blood cells in the blood stream to the fat filled areas of the body.

PHASE 2: The Very Low Calorie Phase (500 cal)

Weigh in the nude, immediately upon wakening, after using the bathroom on the third day. You should have gained at least four pounds during the gorging phase. Inject your fatty tissue. This third day is the first day of Phase 2, the very low calorie phase.

Breakfast is coffee, water, or tea. A tablespoon of fat free milk is permitted. Stevia or saccharin is permitted as well. Drink lots of water during the day, at least a half gallon.

Lunch is 3.5 ounces of red meat, skinless chicken breast, white fleshed fish, or seafood. The seafood allowed is shrimp, scallops, crab, and lobster. Season with most non-caloric seasonings, mustard, apple cider vinegar, lemon, garlic, onions, etc. The foods may be steamed, grilled, broiled, or added to soup broth made from water. The vegetables allowed on Dr. Simeons protocol are green leafy vegetables, tomatoes, onions, fennel, celery, cabbage, red radishes, cucumbers, and asparagus. These may be eaten raw or cooked, as much as fills a regular dinner plate. It is difficult to go over the calorie allotment with vegetables. One grissini style breadstick or one melba toast (plain) is permitted.

For dessert or snack between lunch and dinner, one may eat an apple, a handful of strawberries, or half of one grapefruit.

Dinner is the same regimen, but try to change the vegetables and protein so one gets a variety of nutrients. Vegetables may not be mixed in the same meal.

Weigh in every morning in Phase 2, in the nude after using the restroom, but before anything is taken by mouth. The total calories for the low calorie phase are about 500 daily.

If one stalls in weight loss or gained for three or more days consecutively, a strategy called APPLE DAYS are administered. On these days, measure yourself. Sometimes the scale does not move but the measurements are consistently moving down. If there is no movement of either tool, eat six apples only and just as much water as is necessary to satiate you. The apple days usually result in a loss the next day.

The original protocol was 26 or 43 days including the very low calorie phase and then one moved into Phase 3, without the HCG shots. Transition between Phase 2 and Phase 3 looks like this: the last shot day is called Last Injection Weight, or LIW. Write this number down. One must remain on the 500 calorie plan for the LIW day, followed by two more days. The fourth day one begins Phase 3.

One reason why one loses fat and weight so easily and rapidly on the HCG protocol is because this period of time is a detoxification from unhealthy food choices. The HCG pulls fat from stored fat banks to be used as fuel, so the body still feels like it's receiving about 3000 calories a day. Rather than getting it from your food intake, it is gathered from your own body. The gorging phase ensured that one would have enough fat in the bloodstream, thus turning the appetite off, as well as staving off fatigue when faced with eating 500 calories a day.

PHASE 3: The Stabilization Phase

For three weeks following transition, one adds in more and more calories from other proteins, vegetables, fruits, and healthy fats. Dr. Simeons did not indicate exactly how many calories to take in during this phase, but he did state that absolutely no starches, starchy vegetables or fruits may be taken. Absolutely no sugar may be eaten either. Sugary fruits such as dried fruits, bananas, mangoes, and pineapples are not allowed. In this phase, starchy and sweet vegetables such as carrots, potatoes, sweet winter squashes, and sweet potatoes are not permitted.

The purpose of Phase 3 is to reset the hypothalamus gland into remembering and desiring the newer lower weight as the set point. If Phase 3 is followed correctly, your metabolism will work to stay here instead of returning to the higher weight that the body began from, before the HCG protocol began.

One still weighs in every morning in the nude after elimination. If the scale goes up or down more than two pounds from the LIW, one must commence with a protein day. No food is permitted all day, and then at dinner, one indulges in the largest steak they can eat, along with a large tomato or an apple. That's it. Usually the weight stabilizes itself the next morning. After three weeks of Phase 3, one moves into Phase 4.

PHASE 4: Maintenance Phase

This phase is also three weeks. It is the reintroduction to sugars and starches. For 21 days, try a sugar or a starch one at a time. For example, try bread one day, dried fruit the next day, and jam or a potato the next. If the scale shows more than a two pound gain, this indicates that one is sensitive to that particular food. Write it down and avoid it in the future. Protein days can be used in Phase 4 as well.

A new healthier approach to foods must be followed. It is a lifestyle change. One should eat clean for the most part. The hormone HCG is not approved by the FDA for weight loss because it is very inexpensive. The FDA has approved HCG as a fertility medicine. The diet industry is a multi-billion dollar industry because people fail and have to start the weight loss journey again and again. The HCG protocol is a game changer for the weight and fat loss industry.

The HCG Body for Life protocol modernized the Simeons original protocol and brought it up to date to meet current nutritional profiles for foods. Colin F. Watson is the creator of this revolutionary version. Colin F. Watson's eating plan and books and coaching materials are widely available on the internet. I personally followed his protocol because it simply made more sense to me. I saw the photos of real, individual, long term success stories. The results were not only a thinner body, but a stronger, more muscular, healthy body.

Here are some highlights of the changes Colin F. Watson made when he developed the HCG Body for Life protocol in 2010. He is constantly researching and experimenting in order to make it the most effective for the most number of people.

HCG BODY FOR LIFE OVERVIEW: CHANGES MADE TO THE ORIGINAL SIMEONS' PROTOCOL

PHASE 1: Loading Phase

The loading phase remains the same, but the dosage of the HCG shots or drops have increased to 200 international units per day. From Colin's experiences as a coach, this intake amount seems to have the maximum fat loss while retaining muscle mass.

PHASE 2: The Low Calorie Phase

HCG Body for Life increased the intake of calories to vary between 550-750 per day. Our modern food supply does not have as much nutrition per calorie as it did during Dr. Simeons' era. For example, a fresh apricot today has seven times less vitamins and minerals than it had in 1940, as well as being much larger today, and holds more grams of sugar per ounce. Proteins are also less nutritious and pumped with salt and water. The HCG Body For Life protocol upped the protein values to six ounces of fresh, white-fleshed fish and seafood, close to five ounces of breast meat of chicken, and three and a half ounces of red meat. Exact value guidelines are available on the website,

HCGBODYFORLIFE.COM. Water has been increased to the goal of a gallon of water a day.

Colin added weight bearing exercises to the protocol as well. Muscles burn more calories to maintain themselves than fat, so the more muscles we have and build during the protocol, the more calories burned per day, therefore increasing the metabolism as we lose weight and fat. Colin utilizes high intensity interval training in his guidelines and they are also available for free on YouTube. In Phase 2, when exercising with body resistance or weights, one may go up to 750 calories for that day. Fat free, Greek yogurt may be used as a protein source, being especially effective in fat burning while one sleeps. It is recommended before bed time on those days.

Additional vegetables have been added to the low calorie days. Through his self experimentation and experimenting with family and friends, Colin found that mixing vegetables made the diet more interesting and effective than one vegetable per meal. Mixing vegetables seem beneficial to the nutrient absorption as well. The vegetables added to Phase 2 are zucchini, peppers, mushrooms, broccoli, and Brussels sprouts.

PHASE 3: The Stabilization Phase (3 Weeks)

In Phase 3, the HCG Body For Life protocol eases us into the maximum calorie for our new weight set point. That is the weight on the last injection day. It takes three weeks to do this.

For men, take the last injection weight and multiply that by 12. For women, take the last injection weight and multiply that by 11. That will be the maximum calories allotted for the third week of Phase 3 and beyond. This is when the body is at complete rest, before any exercise calories are burned. If one exercises, and it is highly encouraged, we can eat those burned calories in addition to the base line.

The three weeks look like this for a 180 pound male: 180 x 12 = 2160. That is the maximum calories allotted near the end of Phase 3, before exercise. Take 2160 - 750 = 1410. That is subtracting the low calorie days from the maximum. The 1410 calories extra are divided between the three weeks. 1410 divided by 3 equals 470 calories added each week in Phase 3.

In this example, week one of Phase 3 may have 1220 calories a day plus any calories used in exercise. Week two, this male may have 1690 calories daily plus more if exercising. Week three, this male may have 2160 calories plus any calories burned during physical exercise. Remember to eat more if working out! There are many free applications on the computer and smart phones for tallying the calories in and out. I use My Fitness Pal daily.

The purpose of easing into the maximum calories week by week is to help the weight stabilize within the 2 pound ratio that is so important to maintenance long term. It is also a mental ease, not to shock the body with all those extra calories at the outset of Phase 3.

There is an alternative Phase 3 choice that Colin F. Watson has recently developed. He calls it Phase 3, 2.0. In this Phase 3, the stabilization phase is ten days of very low carbohydrate intake, not more than 30 grams. One must use a nutrient diagnostic program like My Fitness Pal, or something similar, to count net carbohydrate count for the day. The carbohydrate grams minus the fiber grams equal the net carbohydrate grams in any portion of food. When we do this low carbohydrate eating, it turns the body into a fat burner as fuel instead of a sugar burner as fuel. It turns on the ketones in the body, which is the body's mechanism for burning excess body fat as fuel.

The evening of the tenth day, we do carbohydrate back loading. This keeps our body from using muscle tissue as fuel, so the muscles do not atrophy. After the initial ten days, we back load on carbohydrates every five to seven days in the evening. For more information on the entire Phase 3, 2.0 please read the website guidance at www.hcgbodyforlife.com.

PHASE 4: Reintroduction to Starches and Sugars, Maintenance Phase (3 Weeks)

Phase 4 in the HCG Body for Life protocol differs from the Simeons' protocol in this way: Week one, we may add one starch or one sugar at only one meal. Some examples of this are a banana or a piece of toast without jelly. Jelly would be adding a sugar to the starchy bread and this is not permitted in the first week. Pay attention to the scale the next morning. If the weight increases more than two pounds, then that food is probably not good for your particular body, and you are sensitive to it. Write it down, and try to avoid it in the future. Week two of Phase 4, we may add a sugar or a starch to two meals only, but still not in combination. Some examples of this are a banana at breakfast and pasta at dinner. Week three of Phase 4, we may combine sugars and starches in the same meal and see how the body reacts the next morning. Some examples of this are toast with jelly or a piece of cake.

Steak days may be used to regulate the weight in Phase 4 also. If one does not like meat, one may substitute eggs or chicken or fish. The principles are the same as in the original protocol, consuming no food in the day and lots and lots of protein at dinner with an apple or a tomato.

The use of creams and lotions are permitted in HCG Body for Life, unless one deduces that these are the cause of stalls and plateaus during Phase 2. Coconut oil is allowed on the body, and a small amount is permitted for cooking too. The medium chain triglycerides found in coconut oil enhance the weight and fat loss.

Colin eliminated the use of the wheat products in later versions of his protocol. He found it to trigger cravings for starchy carbohydrates and sugars.

The original Dr. Simeons protocol and the HCG Body for Life protocol are both paths to weight and fat loss, a health re-boot, a detoxification, and a time to reflect on why we reach mindlessly for the foods we do. The rapid weight loss is a motivation to keep on going, and the re-setting of the metabolism once finished does make it easier to choose a clean, real food template for life.

Why did I choose this protocol rather than the original? I think of it like I think of the Bible. First came the Old Testament and then came the New Testament. The Old Testament is still valid and beautifully full of prayers and stories that teach us many things. The New Testament is next in line in the history of the ancient texts. It is valid as well and provides us with new hopes and prayers and stories of Divine intervention. Dr. Simeons' original protocol, outlined in his 1954 book, carried the first data of actually curing cases of obesity in the world. It was revolutionary! It is the foundation of the HCG protocol. The HCG Body for Life protocol is simply the successor for the modern human lifestyle.

There are slower methods we can use to lose weight and fat successfully too. I will cover those in later chapters. Whatever method one chooses, make a commitment to that particular protocol. Please don't dabble in this one a little bit, dabble in that one a little bit, sprinkling in some supplements, herbs, and cooking methods from yet a third and fourth lifestyle of eating choices. You won't be able to discern which one is the most effective if you try little bits of many protocols! After you lose the weight and fat, have stabilized for at least six months, feel free to experiment. I have, and am still working through new trials with fat burning and muscle building protocols. If I gain fat and weight to the point where I am not happy with my body composition, then I will turn to the one that worked the most successfully for me, which happens to be HCG Body for Life. Please stay true to your deeper self. When you are quiet for a few moments and stop the insanity of your busy life, you know what works. What works for you may not be what works for everybody. DO YOU, BE YOU.

Now I will share my personal tips and tricks that I discovered during my HCG protocol journey. These things that I stumbled upon made a world of difference in the long run, and every day became more and more fun! The protocol became an adventure, a game, and I intended to win this game! Health miracles do not just fall from the heavens. The right protocol at the right time with the right mind creates those health miracles.

SUPERIOR SELF'S TIPS AND TRICKS FOR HCG AND BEYOND

PRE-PHASE 1: *Getting Ready*

1. Listen to the HCG Body for Life podcasts on iTunes in chronological order. Read the original protocol by Dr. Simeons called *Pounds and Inches: A New Approach to Obesity*. They are both free and available on the internet. Educate yourself as much as possible beforehand so there are less surprises during the phases of the protocol.

2. Ask the meat and fish department at the grocery store to weigh out the protein portions in exact measurements and wrap them separately. Buy at least two week's worth and freeze at home. That way, when you have to hurry off to work, school, appointments, etc., you can simply grab your protein and carry it with you.

3. Order or buy your digital food scale and body scale.

4. Purchase coconut oil, organic, raw, apple cider vinegar, fresh vegetables and fruits, organic when possible. Buy enough produce for a week.

5. Buy cayenne pepper capsules and cinnamon capsules. Buy the strongest mg per capsule that you can find. Buy carnitine tartrate capsules in 500 mg per capsule. These three supplements have helped me tremendously during the low calorie phase of the program, and they have been mentioned in health magazines as being fat burners that actually work in raising metabolism and regulating blood sugar.

6. Buy and start using a body cleanse tablet that begins ten days prior to Phase 1. This cleanses the colon and prepares the body for change.

7. Write down the foods you want to eat in Phase 1, the gorging phase. Write down where you plan to get them, restaurants, bakeries, specialty shops, etc. I say this because as soon as you get the HCG in your system, the appetite goes away! You have to have a game plan to follow in the gorging phase too, even though it sounds silly. When the appetite begins to diminish rapidly, it will be difficult to indulge in those fantasy foods previously eaten without concern. For ultimate success in this program, write everything down and stick to your word! This is your promise to yourself; your word is your bond.

PHASE 1: *The Loading Phase*

1. Take your list of fattening foods and proceed to get them from restaurants, bakeries, and grocery stores. I ate the fattening foods as soon as I returned to my car in order to let it settle while driving to the next location. Treat it like a treasure hunting game, knowing full well that after two days of this game, you will be fed up, literally and figuratively.

2. Do not drink the gallon of water on fat loading days. Drink as much water as is necessary to satisfy thirst. There is less room for food if you are filling up on water.

3. If you can avoid working on gorging days, take those two days off. It is difficult to concentrate while stuffing your face or immediately afterwards. You may not be productive anyway. Plus, people will stare at you if you load correctly. Here you are, already overweight, and then to gorge in front of your coworkers at lunch is sure to raise eyebrows at the very least.

PHASE 2: The Fat Melting Phase

1. When one eats the grapefruit, eat the inside, soft, white, pithy skin and the wax papery looking section separators. This fiber aids greatly in stool regularity.

2. Take a good quality multivitamin, cayenne pepper capsules, and cinnamon capsules before retiring at night. They may be harsh on the stomach but by the time they hit your tummy, you are asleep, so chances are you won't know it. The carnitine tartrate capsules may be taken any time of the day or evening. I continue taking ten of each supplement daily, even now. The company called Nutrabio sells pharmaceutical grade carnitine tartrate without fillers or binders on their website. Of all of the fat burners and sugar regulators in the world, these three supplements have been indicated to be effective. My personal experience with these fat burners has been consistent. When I don't take these three supplements for three weeks, I feel less strong and I look softer rather than leaner.

3. Drink apple cider vinegar shots or put the shots in a glass of water and chug it. It tastes very sour and wakes us up!! Use it in salads and soups

for flavoring. The apple cider vinegar kills sugar cravings and creates an alkaline environment in the body. This is an anti-inflammatory, aids in digestion, and in fat burning too.

4. Add herbs, lemon, or cucumber slices to your water. Drink water all day and night, hot or cold. The added fruit and herb essences in the water helped me get the gallon of water into my body. It was a challenge at first, but in about ten days to two weeks, you will become acclimated to the amount of water taken in.

5. Chewing on real cinnamon sticks is like sucking on spicy candy all day long. Cinnamon gets sweeter the longer you suck and chew on it. It kills sugar cravings, and makes your teeth look whiter too!

6. Keep canned crab (in water) in your car, desk, backpack, locker, purse, etc. The can is perfect for travel and is a great portion size to top onto salads or cooked vegetables. Just add lemon and seasoning. Don't forget the can opener!

7. Carry your pre-portioned frozen protein in a ziploc bag. Take it with you anywhere. In a

pinch, when you don't have access to a stove, it is easy to place in a bowl and microwave for a few minutes for cooking with seasoning. Now you have a moist or soupy protein to eat quickly with your greens!

8. Lakanto golden variety is a sugar substitute that looks, tastes, and smells like brown sugar. This is the only natural sweetener I found to be authentic to the sugar flavor profile. It is zero on the glycemic index and is zero calories. It is made from the Chinese monk fruit called luo han gao. It has been used for thousands of years in Asia for a variety of ailments. This natural sweetener is readily available on line. Xyla is a natural white sugar substitute. It is made from xylitol, originally from the birch tree and other barks. It has 9 calories per teaspoon and is really hard to tell from white table sugar! Both of these sugar substitutes may be used in the ratio of 1 to 1 instead of regular sugar.

9. Probiotics found in naturally fermented foods aid digestion and elimination. I found raw sauerkraut, kimchi, and vinegar in all forms to be extremely helpful in regulating my bowel movements.

10. Black Pu-erh tea, which is an extra aged fermented tea from China, has been shown to aid in increased metabolism. Green tea in excess of eight cups a day has been shown to do so also.

11. Aloe vera juice helps with elimination of foods through the system. Pure unsweetened aloe vera juice has zero calories and is sold by the gallon at drugstores nationwide.

12. Kale has high quality protein and is highly filling. I rub chopped kale leaves with coconut oil, Himalayan salt, and spices. Then I lay the mixture on a cookie sheet lined with parchment paper. I bake at 375 degrees for about 20 minutes, turning often. Think about them as a kind of potato chip for Phase 2 and beyond. My children even prefer them over potato chips now! Fresh or dried seaweed without oil is a high source of iodine and fiber too. Some of the vegetables I eat during Phase 2 weren't available to a wide audience in Europe in the 1940s, 1950s, and 1960s, when Dr. Simeons developed and wrote his protocol. Nowadays there are many more low calorie, nutrient dense, water filled vegetables that won't compromise your HCG weight loss. Colin F.

Watson and I have done the experimenting for you! Take our word for it.

13. If struggling with emotional impulses to eat something not on protocol, take a deep breath, close your eyes, and clench both fists as tightly as possible. With clenched fists, say to yourself, "I love myself more than I love this food." Say this ten times out loud while keeping the fists clenched the entire time. Then walk away from the food and fill a mug with hot water with lemon. Drink this immediately. I can't tell you how many times this tool saved me from falling off of the wagon!

14. If at a stall or a gain in Phase 2, take a hot epsom salt bath with a lot of baking soda for at least twenty minutes. This also helps during menstruation or if feeling bloated.

15. Nutritional yeast is a natural fungus that has low calories, lots of B vitamins for energy, and is a great protein source. It is fat free, gluten free, sugar free, and carbohydrate free. It has 8 grams of protein for two tablespoons. The best thing about nutritional yeast for me is that it tastes like grated parmesan cheese. I sprinkle it on vegetables, proteins, and salads.

16. Great Lakes unflavored powdered gelatin is a wonderful source of fat free protein. It adds protein to any liquid and has no flavor! One tablespoon has 25 calories and 6 grams of protein. It can also thicken soups and gravies.

17. Healthy 'n' Fit brand 100 percent egg protein is a non-chalky tasting protein powder. I am very hard to please with any powder and I think the vanilla ice cream flavor really is good, with no artificial sweeteners! They use stevia to sweeten it. One scoop has 100 calories and 24 grams of protein. I add it to water and ice for an ice cream smoothie that is good for me.

18. If at a function that is unavoidable, such as a work party, business luncheon, seminar, convention, or family and friend celebration, declare an apple day. This takes all the stress out of figuring out what you can eat or not eat at the party. When people begin to ask you why you are not partaking in the goodies, just say you are on a restricted diet right now. That way the guilt and embarrassment will be taken out of the equation, and most folks won't pry into it any further. It leaves the whole story sharing situation up to you, when you are comfortable

or close enough to your goal to be divulging the details of your journey.

19. Restaurants that you can eat at during this phase are Japanese for raw white fleshed fish (sashimi), or a buffet place that has raw vegetables, salads without dressings, and grilled fish or meats that you can see them cook. Many Asian buffet style restaurants are Phase 2 friendly. I am good enough now to eyeball the ounces, but feel free to bring your digital food scale and gluten free tamari sauce.

20. Track your food intake on a free program or application such as My Fitness Pal. It really does break down every ingredient, caloric value, and balance of the fat to protein to carbohydrate ratio. It has been an invaluable tool to see a diary of every little thing passing my lips and not marrying my hips!

PHASE 3: The Stabilization Phase

1. Canned fish in water, mustard, or brine have become a staple in my car. Sardines, clams, oysters, anchovies, trout, mackerel, tuna, and kipper snacks are available for rock bottom

prices. Some varieties I even find at the dollar store. I take them everywhere in case I can't find healthy protein options on the go. I can't be sure of what kinds of oils are used in the preparation of my food in a restaurant unless it is sashimi in a Japanese restaurant (no oil at all).

2. Quest bars are protein bars made with 20 grams of bioavailable protein. That means the body can absorb and use what it is inside of the bar, rather than just digesting it through the body to be eliminated as waste. All flavors are sugar free and a great many of them are made with stevia and luo han gao (Chinese monk fruit). Quest bars are gluten free and grain free. They are high fiber and have very low carbohydrate totals, very low on the glycemic index. This is the only brand that I found not to taste chalky to me. They are also low fat. The calories range from 160-210, depending on the flavor. These dessert alternatives can be found at GNC or on the internet.

3. Measure out one ounce portions of raw tree nuts, and keep in baggies around the house or in the car. They provide smart fats which satiate the appetite for longer periods of time. Roasted and salted tree nuts change the molecules of

fat, therefore making it easier to overeat them. Roasted nut oils become the type of fat that is not as healthy for us. The right kinds of dietary fat do not become fat on our body.

4. Pure Protein brand of milk shakes are available in a can. I like the 35 gram protein can, vanilla cream flavor. It has only one gram of sugar per can, and this is not added cane sugar. It has only a few grams of carbohydrates and actually tastes great. I am sensitive to most protein shakes and powders, having a hard time with the chalkiness texture. I usually get a gag reflex. This brand is not only one that I can tolerate, but enjoy.

5. Alligator meat is virtually fat free! If you can find it where you live, buy it. Three and a half ounces of this super food has 50 grams of protein and 232 calories. It is a very concentrated source of protein.

6. Raw chocolate and raw cacao nibs contain good fats and antioxidants. It also releases euphoric sensations in the brain. It raises good cholesterol and lowers bad cholesterol. I make my own chocolate treats by adding raw nuts, coconut oil, shredded raw coconut, cinnamon, Lakanto, and raw unpasteurized cream.

7. Fresh coconut pieces are delicious when baked in the oven for an hour on 350 degrees. I add heavy shakes of Lakanto and cinnamon before baking.

8. Raw unpasteurized dairy products have helped me add good fats into my life without fear. It brought back my feminine roundness in my breasts and buttocks without adding any weight!

9. Ground flax seeds and chia seeds that are soaked for 15 minutes help balance the Omega oils 3-6-9 in our diet. I add them to my water bottle with lemon, electrolyte powder, and green veggie and fruit powder from Trader Joes or the Institute For Vibrant Living.

10. Continue to consume a gallon of water a day, as it helps to keep us full as our bodies get used to normal hunger patterns without the HCG in our systems.

PHASE 4: The Maintenance Phase

Phase 4 can be quite scary. You have gone at least 47 days without starchy carbohydrates and sugars. You have lost weight and fat, all the while keeping muscle mass. You have detoxified the body of artificial flavors, preservatives and chemicals. You have eaten a colorful array of extremely healthy vegetables, fruits, and protein sources. You have given up "white" foods.

Now, to begin adding back in sugars and starches little by little can be daunting. We are at the maximum caloric intake at this point in the protocol. We may add more calories in if we burn calories by daily activities and exercise.

The first week of Phase 4, I chose to try sugars rather than starches because I missed sweet things more than savory foods. Surprising to me, ice cream (home churned, of course), chocolate, and dried fruit did not affect my weight.

The second week of Phase 4, I tried sugars and starches, separately, but I only felt comfortable doing this at one meal per day, even though HCG Body for Life allows it up to two times a day.

Week three of Phase 4 was the real mental challenge for me. I was petrified when I ate a flaky pastry with cheese and preserves inside of it. I did not gain an ounce! The next few days I remained stable with my weight. The sixth day of my last week in Phase 4, I chose a half cup of white rice with my salad (no dressing) and grilled fish. The next day I was two pounds up! Message to self: my body doesn't do well with white rice.

I realized through trial and error during Phase 4 that the stress and worry of seeing if the scale would go up a few pounds after a sugary item or a starchy item just was not worth it for me. I decided to live on Phase 3 foods permanently, and use sugary or starchy foods as a treat. For my mental clarity and ease of living, this was my personal solution. I encourage you to do what feels right and relaxed for *you* in Phase 4 and beyond. When one feels stressed out all of the time, it creates cortisol to be released into the body and this holds us in emergency mode, holding on to the fat instead of using it as energy.

Basically, I am living my life as though I am a diabetic person with celiac disease. I do not have these diseases but it is an easier meal template for me to live with. I flow through life easily now with the preparation of meals for myself and my family. I did not realize that living grain free and sugar free was called Paleo, Ancestral, Primal, and Evolutionary. It took me almost two years to evolve into a mostly organic, mostly grain free, mostly sugar free individual. I practice very clean eating ninety percent of the time. The other ten percent I party like a rock star without guilt or negative self-judgment. My body knows how to recover after a treat day because the healthy learned habits are fully ingrained into my daily life. A balanced, relatively low carbohydrate lifestyle, with low glycemic index foods are my norm, keeping my body in balance with sustained energy.

I use sugar free calcium chews and gummy vitamins as alternatives to candy. I love Lulu's raw chocolates, made with coconut crystals instead of sugar. It has all of the great antioxidants that organic dark chocolates provide, without fillers, binders, soy, or sugar. Recently I discovered an organic Venezuelan chocolate paste called Ek-Chok. It is sugar free and oh-so satisfying. It also utilizes coconut crystals instead of sugar.

Throughout Phase 4, if I discovered a carbohydrate source or a sugary product that made me gain weight the morning after, I would write it down on an index card. A good idea is to keep the card taped to the inside of a kitchen cupboard. Allow it to be a guide to what does not work for your personal body chemistry, your trigger foods, and things that you are sensitive to, even though you may not be allergic to them.

Food sensitivities and food allergies are not the same thing. Allergies occur in the blood stream. Sensitivities occur in the stomach or intestines. Allergies can have a dramatic reaction that can sometimes be dangerous or even deadly. Sensitivities are usually milder and can resemble "normal" aches, pains, acne, flu, or cold symptoms. If I suffered from a rash, stomach pain, diarrhea, or back pain right after ingesting a particular food that I could identify, I would avoid it for a while. Then to make certain that the food in question was or was not the culprit, I would try it again. Sometimes our food sensitivities change over time and we can eat what previously made us feel discomfort.

Eating food that causes me headaches or stomach pain will make me eat it less often. It definitely has an impact on me, but I will indulge once in a while even though I know the discomfort that comes later. Humans naturally attempt to avoid pain. If a respected mentor tells me that the food in question will make me fat, I will give it up entirely. The word *fat* is a trigger for most people. I will have forbidden foods now and then, fully knowing the consequences, but say the F word, and I am done with it forever!

In Phase 4, I focused on remembering that I am a spirit on a human journey and I chose to have this human challenge of optimum health and wellness. I loved myself a little more each day, each time that

I reached for something nutritious and life giving. Moving closer to my true self was *me*, moving in a positive direction. I could not turn back now. Phase 4 had taken me so far from my former choices. I encourage you to love yourself a little bit more during the last three weeks of the protocol, rather than beat yourself up mentally or feel guilty if you eat something that resulted in a gain. It is just information, not a judgement call.

The HCG protocol is a systematic way to successfully change one's habits for life. It is not called a diet because it is not intended for one to return to the previous methods of eating afterwards. It is a complete lifestyle change that once embraced whole heartedly, can assist in whole person wellness and not just thinness. Our way of viewing food will change. Our way of viewing who we truly are will improve.

Chapter Four

WHAT I EAT NOW
(AND WHAT
I DON'T)

*A*fter the HCG journey was completed, the journey of who I am, and what I wanted to do with the relatively short process became evident almost immediately. I discovered podcasts, articles, magazines, books, lectures, and radio shows that challenged me to become aware of even more health and wellness facts. There were a couple of years of gradual layers of learning, where I took notes daily from the media and from my personal experimentation. I began coaching others on their wellness path too. I was burning with desire to learn as much information as possible, to reach as many people as possible.

What do incredibly healthy people all have in common? Radiant energy. We sense it when they are in our personal space. I decided to assist others to stop settling for their life the way it is, and to truly start living for themselves on a higher level.

Our bodies seamlessly know what to do and have all the answers if we humans get out of our own way. We are so brain smart and forward thinking that we have forgotten the basic ways we have lived for eons before processed foods, raspberry ketones, Garcinia Cambogia, point counting, calorie counting, and green coffee bean extract came onto the scene. Before all the fad diets and potions, we humans thrived rather than survived. We radiated energy, and functioned without modern conveniences quite well, thank you. Funny thing is, nowadays we have to schedule and plan ahead our methods of simplification. I'm with you there. I need to strategize my food shopping to get the raw veggies, healthy raw fats, raw pastured dairy, pastured eggs, and proteins from specific specialty stores all over San Francisco. Strategic planning and action firmly sets our intention in place. My thoughts gravitate towards completing my to-do list. Then I feel so accomplished at finishing my to-do list, I am happy to reap the rewards by partaking in the cooking and eating of the things I so painstakingly procured!

Results are a happy smiling me, which results in a happy smiling husband and kids. Radiance. If I grabbed takeout food or drive through pickups on my busy day, the result would be a crabby me, nutrient poor delivery of foods to the cells in my body, a bad attitude, acne, gas, weight fluctuations, and a general lackluster life. Not radiant.

Food and workouts are a part of it, as well as a spiritual path. So many people put their focus on the calories burned during a workout. Yes, working out in any form is awesome, but it is only part of a holistic approach. What are we doing the other hours of the day? How are we recovering from the exercise? What we do with the other hours that we are not exercising is far more important than what we do for the duration of the physical exertion. The recovery time can ruin your efforts or support your efforts.

After my HCG journey was complete, I had to relearn that calories do not matter as much as the quality of the food I was eating. Our bodies adapt to whatever amount of food we give it. If I eat healthy and high fat, good quality fat, I will have lots of energy to be more active and burn off those calories of food. If I starve myself I will feel lethargic, and my output of energy will reduce to match what I put into the body.

Our bodies are way smarter than our minds. It is not just simple math. So, what do I eat now, and what do I encourage others to embrace as part of their holistic approach to food? What do I stay away from?

We must first stop thinking of food as a reward or a punishment, in any sense of those definitions. We are not good or bad people as a result of eating! We are just eating. Food is sustenance. Food is fuel. Our goodness as human beings is a separate thing entirely. I'm not saying that food is not enjoyable or pleasurable or fun, even. It is, and it should be. I am saying that one hundred percent focus on food one hundred percent of the time does not work for us, unless we are in culinary school or working as a chef in the industry.

This chapter will give you some basic information about **grains, fats, sugar, probiotics, raw dairy, and proteins**. It goes without saying that chemicals and artificial ingredients are pretty much not part of my daily routine. I will also share my motto for *maintenance* of the weight and fat loss. Let's start there.

A long time ago my husband told me of the three Ds:

- **Desire**
- **Determination**
- **Dedication**

These **D** words have morphed over the years to become a family mantra. They hold great meaning to me in spelling out success in health, fitness, and other life goals.

Desire is the end result goal that one wants. State it and write it down. Say it loud and say it proud! This is your future calling!

Determination is the process that one goes through in order to make that happen. Once the steps are revealed as to what to do, stick to it and follow the steps in order.

Dedication is the commitment one has to seeing the whole thing through to the finish line.

Together these three Ds spell out success. The three Ds can be used for reaching for your superior self. Challenge yourself with new health, fitness, mind, and spiritual quests. Follow the three Ds by writing it all down, and then GO!

The more I experimented with ancestral, primal, Paleolithic, evolutionary, non-starch, and non- sugar eating patterns, the healthier and happier I became! Funny thing, all things old become new and fashionable again, not just in fashion and beauty, but in nutrition too. Rapidly, I gave up all grain products and animals that ate grains. My cravings for sweets were replaced by cravings for fats.

I naturally and effortlessly became accustomed to unplanned intermittent fasting, which furthers fat burning. It turns the body into a fat burning machine. I never get hungry now from dinner one evening to about 2pm the next day. I tried vegetable juice fasting for a week and the result was a renewed awareness of how sweet food can be, even when it is just vegetables! I also learned fake hunger versus true hunger signals. The clock no longer dictates when I eat. My true hunger does.

True hunger is difficult to gauge when we are bombarded with commercials and magazine ads telling us of some new must-have convenience foods. 100 calorie packs, heart healthy, whole grain, fat free, all natural...Buzz words like these show us that we are not intelligent enough to make our own decisions based on the truth. No wonder we are so confused! The people on those television ads look so happy, healthy, thin, and fit drinking soda and chips!

GRAINS

Simply put, humans are not meant to eat grains and processed grains. Just think of the oats growing in the wild. How much work is it to process the inedible natural grain to make it digestible by the body as oatmeal? A LOT. Yes, there have been grains in the human diet for about ten thousand years. But for millions of years before that, we humans did not eat grains. The genetically altered grains of today are very different from the ancient grains of our past. They soaked the grains overnight to become soft enough to be used in any form or fashion. Gluten is the protein in the wheat, rye, and barley that make it fluffy and help things rise when baking. It gives baked items a chewy and fluffy texture. It can make us fluffy too.

Grain products naturally increase blood sugar and inflammation in the body. Increased blood sugar and inflammation can contribute to weight gain, blood pressure problems, swings in energy and mood, and a host of other inflammatory chronic diseases. It creates in the body a level of discomfort, a kind of *dis-ease.* These symptoms, if left unchecked, may lead to disease. It is not rocket science.

We can also reverse this. The lack of grains and grain products in one's diet may lead to the relief or cure of many of these ailments. In my own experience, I have no more gas pains, bloating, or joint pain since giving up grains. When on the rare occasion that I do indulge in a grain product, I immediately get a headache that lasts for about twenty four hours. I am not a person who gets headaches at all! In fact, I used to tease my kids that if Mama got a headache, stay far away from me because I would soon have the flu for three weeks, and was probably contagious. I can now see my abdominal muscles as I exercise, not just when on the losing phase of a protocol. I have said goodbye to constipation. The remarkable thing about refraining from grains is that I noticed the improvements in about thirty days.

FATS

The brain is more than two thirds fat, so when we do not take in enough healthy, good-for-us dietary fats, our body is out of balance, out of homeostasis. The imbalance can cause forgetfulness and depression. This cognitive decline is commonly called brain fog. Our body needs fats that will be readily absorbed into the bloodstream. This ability to be absorbed and used well by the body is called bioavailability. The fats that are well absorbed also aid in the absorption of the vitamins and minerals of the foods eaten alongside of them.

After losing the weight on the HCG Body for Life protocol, I added healthy fats back into my diet. The roundness in my cheeks, buttocks, and breasts quickly returned. After three weeks of coconut flakes, avocado, raw butter, raw nuts, ghee, and raw cheeses in small quantities, I had more energy and glowed. People began asking questions about my skincare regime. I was working on the skincare routine from the inside out, with water and fat.

Remembering my elementary school science, it made sense. Fat floats on top, so my skin appeared more full, soft, and fatty, but in a good way! Remember, fat does not make us fat, if it is the right kind of fat. I now eat fifty to seventy five percent of my daily caloric intake from fat. I track it on my computer or smart phone with My Fitness Pal. There are many free applications available to assist in the nutrient balance of your food intake.

We should eat fats from:

- COCONUT
- AVOCADO
- OLIVES
- RAW NUTS AND SEEDS
- RAW NUT AND SEED BUTTERS/OILS
- GRASS FED BUTTER AND GHEE
- GRASS FED RAW BUTTER
- GRASS FED RAW DAIRY PRODUCTS
- GRASS FED, GRASS FINISHED ANIMALS
- 100% PASTURED EGGS

Coconut

Coconut oil was given a bad rap for so long in the mainstream medical communities because it is a saturated fat. Saturated fat used to be blamed for heart disease, and it is very difficult to rid the mind of old dogma. Saturated fat is a fat that gets solidified at room temperature or cooler. Coconut milk, oil, and flesh has recently been redeemed from the "bad" fat list. The fatty acids in coconut products help us absorb minerals like calcium, magnesium, and boron from other foods. This is important for maintaining strong bones.

Coconut oil is made up of medium chain fatty acids which get used immediately by the body as energy instead of being converted into fat molecules on our hips, thighs, and abdomens. Coconut oil also helps our body to balance the Omega 3 and Omega 6 oils. This assists the body in using the stored fat on our hips, thighs, and abdomens as energy for everyday living.

Coconut products reduce internal stress, kill bad bacteria, aid in curing inflammation, inflammatory diseases, and it is a natural anti-viral. Coconut has been used around the world for centuries as both food and medicine.

I use coconut oil daily on my hair, skin, and nails. I throw it in the bath. I swish with it for fifteen minutes three times a week as a teeth whitener and gum strengthener. I cook with it, bake with it, and oil the furniture with it. In the HCG Body for Life protocol, it was the only fat allowed during Phase 2, the low calorie phase. It did not cause fat loss stalls or plateaus. When I bake desserts, I use coconut flour and oil as a substitute for other oils and flours. The results are wonderful! I even make coconut based ice cream. I drink fresh coconut water when available. In fact, in certain parts of the Philippines, they use coconut water in an IV when blood for blood transfusions aren't available. As soon as it hits the blood stream, the coconut water changes into blood molecules.

Avocado

Avocado is used as a liver detoxification tool in many countries. It is a fatty fruit which has monounsaturated fats in it. They are helpful for reducing bad cholesterol, reducing cancer risk and diabetes risk. People who consume lots of avocados usually have lower fat percentages in their whole body ratio. Oh, did I mention it is delicious?

Olives

Olives are another source of healthy, monounsaturated fats. Like the avocado, it is considered a fruit because it comes from a tree. The olive and olive oils contain long chain fatty acids. When buying olive oil, a good idea is to purchase authentic extra virgin olive oil. Many labeled extra virgin olive oils in our stores are not the real thing, and are sometimes blended with a lower quality olive oil. Make sure to buy one that is certified organic, with a harvest date stamped on the back of the bottle or can. These are the least processed kinds of olive oil.

Olive oil is best utilized by the body at room temperature instead of cooking with it. When olive oil gets heated beyond its smoke point, the chemical components of the oil break down and the oil becomes toxic. Room temperature olive oil can lower the risk of heart disease by reducing the LDL cholesterol. The LDL cholesterol is the "bad" cholesterol. There are anti-oxidants in the olive oil which protect cells from the damage we incur when we don't eat well (or drink well!). Olives and olive oil have vitamin K in it, second only to green leafy vegetables. Olives and olive oil are considered functional food. A functional food is easily absorbed by the body (bioavailable) and helps with multiple benefits beyond its basic nutrition.

Raw Nuts and Seeds, Their Butters and Oils

I consume loads of raw nuts and seeds. Why raw? When roasted, the oil in them becomes changed and the potential to harm health rather than enhance health is increased as the temperature increases in the nuts and seeds. Sticking to the raw form seems to avoid potential problems. For me, raw nuts and seeds are difficult to overeat. I feel fuller on raw versus roasted, and the fat content keeps me satisfied way longer than when I eat roasted nuts. I can speed-eat roasted nuts, and if they are salted, it is a danger zone for me. Raw nuts and seeds contain balances between Omega fats 3-6-9, and are a wonderful source of protein, fiber, and amino acids (the building blocks of proteins). They contain a variety of vitamins and minerals, are delicious, and very satisfying to the palate.

I use cold-pressed, organic oils from hemp seeds, grape seeds, sesame seeds, macadamia nuts, walnuts, and avocados. Surprising to me, hemp seed oil cured my acne when applied topically to my skin. Even old scars faded for me rather quickly. Hemp seeds are a plant source that have a complete protein profile. They contain all six essential amino acids and are bioavailable to the body. These oils mentioned here are freely available at Asian supermarkets and on the internet at health food discount companies.

I purchase MCT oil on the internet too. I use it to boost up my energy before a long night of serving food and drink at the restaurant where I work. MCT oil is the best part of the fat from the coconut mixed with the best part of the red palm and camphor trees. Together they form a kind of super food. They aid in the digestion of other food nutrients and absorption of essential vitamins and minerals. MCT oil helps us to naturally fast. Many hours pass before I get hungry again after using MCT oil. MCT stands for medium chain triglycerides, which I mentioned earlier in the coconut section of this chapter. MCT oil assists in the burning of body fat while maintaining lean muscle mass.

Raw nut and seed butters are my favorite sweet treat when I am craving dessert (PMS, anyone?). I add a few tablespoons to my nonfat Greek yogurt, toss in Lakanto, cinnamon, and shredded, dry, raw coconut. Sometimes I add a tablespoon of powdered bee pollen. Mmmmm, good. Raw nut and seed butters still have the fiber and protein in it, whereas the oils have just the fat. Read your labels! The lower number of ingredients a food product has, the better the nutritional values. If you see very scientific, hard to read words in the ingredients list, chances are that the company who made the nut and seed butters added things in that you do not want in your body.

A word about peanuts: Peanuts are not a nut at all. They are a bean, part of the legume family. They grow underground, like many beans, whereas nuts grow on trees. Unlike tree nuts, peanuts are better absorbed by the body when they are roasted instead of raw. They should be roasted on a low setting in the oven, a little below 200 degrees Fahrenheit, for about fifteen to twenty minutes, turning often. This helps them to be digested and kills any invisible molds on the peanuts' surface. There is no need to add oil, as they contain oil which rises to the surface when baked. Peanuts are higher in Omega 6 oils than other nuts, which in excess can be considered a bad fat, so I eat them sparingly. It is also higher in carbohydrates than other nuts.

Butter, Raw Butter, and Ghee

Butter that is from cows who only eat grass is called pastured butter. It helps us absorb the nutrients in foods that we eat with it. If it is raw butter, that means it has not been heated at all or pasteurized. This is even healthier. Sometimes when I know that I am not going to be able to take a break from serving at the restaurant where I work,

I will eat a few tablespoons of raw butter, mixed with raw nuts, Lakanto, and cinnamon just before my shift. It does keep me satiated and energized so I don't reach for junk that won't feed my nutritional needs. I used to reach for unhealthy snacks back in the day. I know that you know exactly what I mean. I feel you nodding through the pages, shaking your head in agreement.

Ghee is a type of clarified butter, golden yellow in color. It is made by cooking the grass fed butter and removing the thick bubbly residue that floats on the top. The good fat stays and the milk residue is removed. Ghee needs no refrigeration after this process and is another great source of healthy saturated fat. Ghee has a higher smoke point than butter too, so it is ideal for cooking even at high heats. Ghee originated in India. I remember being in India, and watching the women hand feed their dogs ghee and rice and chapati (flat, round, whole wheat breads). The dogs in India had the shiniest fur coats ever!

Raw Dairy

Raw milk and raw cheeses from unpasteurized milk and cream are beneficial and delicious. There are more and more stores selling unpasteurized dairy products than ever before. If someone is lactose intolerant, they still may be able to enjoy raw dairy because the lactase enzyme has not been changed into lactose through the pasteurization process. Raw milk products provided from grass fed animals provide protein, fat, and calcium to the body. Calcium is more easily metabolized by the bones when compared to pasteurized dairy. I think if humans were lactase intolerant, they could not easily nurse on their mothers' milk. Humans lactate.

Grass Fed Animals

The skin and fat found on 100% grass fed and grass finished animals are extremely healthy for our skin and organs. Omega 3 fats, which are great for brain health are found in higher amounts in 100% grass fed and grass finished animals. The fatty organ meats are also very nutritious. Sometimes organ meats are difficult to get used to if one has not grown up with it in their family's diet. People may be unsure of how to cook them. Personally, I usually don't eat red meat, but I do love chicken livers and chicken skin from my pastured chickens. Pastured chicken means that the chicken was never fed any grains in its life. It roamed the farm or field and only consumed plants, bugs, berries, or other fruit that fell to the ground. The easiest way for me to enjoy organ meats is to sauté them with lots of garlic, onions, leeks, turmeric, and butter.

Pastured Eggs

Likewise, the eggs in my refrigerator are from 100% pastured chickens. They sure are expensive, but worth it to me. If you eat an animal, you eat what the animal ate. So if you eat a grain fed animal, it has the potential to cause the same reaction in the body as if you ate grains. I'm not willing to back to square one with that. I have come so far and am so much healthier now.

Fats that I stay away from are trans-fats. Trans-fats are toxic to the body in large quantities. Examples of trans-fats are shortening, margarine, and any processed oil that has been made to stay hard at room temperature. This helps foods stay on the grocery store shelves longer without spoiling. Omega 6 oils in highly processed vegetable oils should be avoided as well. Examples of Omega 6 oils are soy, corn, cotton seed, canola, peanut, sunflower, and safflower oils. Trans-fats raise LDL, the bad cholesterol, and lower HDL, the good cholesterol. Omega 6 oils are inflammatory in nature. Omega 6 oils are often made into trans-fats by processing, and then strategically placed into highly refined, packaged foods. For me, it is reasonably easy to avoid trans-fats because they are usually found combined with processed grain products, which I avoid like the plague anyway. If one indulges in sources of Omega 6 fatty acid foods or trans-fats, be certain to have plenty of healthy Omega 3 oils as well, like in fatty fish, seafood, and the saturated good fats mentioned earlier. They will balance out the ratio of "good" to "bad" fats.

SUGAR

There are many names for sugar, and I strive to steer clear of them all! Once in a while I will make a conscious choice to indulge, with no guilt. Here are some common names for sugar:

- AGAVE
- BARLEY MALT
- BEET SUGAR
- CANE JUICE
- EVAPORATED CANE SYRUP
- HONEY
- DATE SUGAR
- FRUCTOSE
- LACTOSE
- MALTOSE
- RICE SYRUP
- TURBINADO SUGAR
- HIGH FRUCTOSE CORN SYRUP

There are many more than these listed here. I find them added in to most packaged foods. Please note here that I am not referring to the sugar naturally found in fruits and vegetables. In their whole form, fruits and vegetables have fiber and vitamins bound to them. That is wonderful news to the body.

Carbohydrates and sugar both turn to glucose sugar when it hits the blood stream as it is absorbed from food. Sugar releases feel-good hormones in the brain, making it an easy substance to get addicted to.

Our first meal as newborns was incredibly sweet. Mothers' milk or formula is sickeningly sweet. Have you ever tasted it as an adult? Yuck! I find it too sweet. We are hard wired to love sweet things. Add to that the emotional bonds created early in life. When nursing on our mothers' breasts or being fed formula at a close proximity to the ones we love the most, it is understandable why we continue the sweets addiction throughout our lives. Milestones are celebrated with sweet things: weddings, birthdays, anniversaries, holidays, religious ceremonies, etc.

Take a look at an ice cream shop on a hot day. There are lines around a block! Now take a look at a produce shop on the very same day. I'm pretty certain that there will be plenty of room for me, and no wait in line either. What is it about sugar that we so adore?

Well, besides the sweet childhood memories, they provoke pleasure hormones in the brain. Glucose is necessary for the body to function, but it doesn't have to come from the sugar added to foods. Our body can make its own glucose. It can even convert protein into glucose if it needs to, or if we eat way more protein than we need to survive the day, the excess will be converted into glucose. Our bodies' capabilities are remarkable.

The sugar that is added to most packaged foods disturbs the body's homeostasis. Sugar pulls minerals from the body where they are needed most and continued abuse messes up the body chemistry. Eventually this affects immunity and makes us ill, or more susceptible to becoming ill. Sugar feeds cancer cells very efficiently, and can neutralize any good changes that chemotherapy may provide.

When we eat a large quantity of our diet from starchy carbohydrates and sugar, we cause the insulin to work improperly, hence creating a broken metabolism. A broken metabolism resulted in my weight gain and joint pain. I was lucky though. I was able to run sixteen marathons with a broken metabolism. Others aren't so lucky.

If the insulin receptors malfunction, fat is stored rather than used. The dam of good health may be broken and a variety of illnesses may ensue: obesity, type 2 diabetes, brain fog, hormonal imbalances, fatigue, digestive issues, mental issues, and an increase in cancer susceptibility. That's just the beginning of my list!

Our entire body has only 5 grams of sugar floating around in the blood stream at any one time. Five grams! That's a teaspoon! How much sugar is in one bowl of "heart-healthy," whole grain cereal? There are way more than 5 grams. What is our body supposed to do with the other grams of sugar that we feed it? If we aren't immediately doing high, intense cardiovascular exercise or intensive weight training, our body has no choice but to store it as fat to be used later on as energy. Do this enough...that is, eat whole grain cereals and sugar daily, and it may be easy to upset the hormonal balance, become overweight, and show symptoms of illnesses that go along with obesity.

Let's look at the typical breakfast, lunch, and dinner of the Standard American Diet: Breakfast includes cereal, fruit, and juice. Lunch includes a sandwich, salad with dressing from a bottle, and a cookie. Dinner includes a meat or fish, a starch, and a vegetable. Add rolls and butter, sometimes alcohol, and sometimes dessert. Every meal in the example of the Standard American Diet has more than the 5 grams of sugar that we can easily handle floating around in our bloodstream. This, to me, is a clear recipe for a health disaster. No wonder our medical system thrives upon sick care and not preventive care!

So, what do I do to satisfy my sweet tooth? Women seem to be attracted to desserts more than men, although that's not an absolute. My cravings are stronger right before and during the beginning of my menstruation. I use Lakanto golden brown sugar substitute. I love it so much and mention it to people all the time on my blog. It is made from Luo Han Guo, a Chinese monk fruit. It is zero calories, zero on the glycemic index, and best of all to me, it has no weird chemical aftertaste. I enjoy the golden brown variety the best, although they have a white sugar style sweetener as well. Lakanto looks, tastes, and smells like real brown sugar. It acts like real sugar in recipes. As of now, Lakanto is available on the internet only. It is very expensive, but worth it to me in order to maintain my healthy lifestyle.

For baking and sugary needs at a lesser cost, there is a product I like called Xyla. It is xylitol, made from birch bark. It is crystalized like white sugar, is used like white sugar in baking, recipes, and in your coffee, tea, etc. It even sparkles like white sugar. It is low on the glycemic index, but it does have about 9 calories per teaspoon. Xyla can be found in health food stores, higher quality grocery stores, and on the internet.

Stevia is a good all natural plant alternative to sugar. Be sure to read the ingredients on the stevia package. Some companies add corn starch to their product during the powdering process. This makes the product last longer on the shelves and is a cheaper alternative to pure stevia. To me, stevia has a funny aftertaste similar to chemical artificial sweeteners. Some folks outgrow the sensitivity. I never have, so I use the above mentioned sweeteners instead.

For my sugar free chocolate cravings, I turn to Lulu's Raw chocolate. These small bars are raw and organic. They use coconut crystals instead of sugar, also extremely low on the glycemic index. Raw chocolate has loads of good fats and antioxidants. Sometimes I make my own chocolates with raw cacao nibs or powder, coconut oil, raw butter, raw cream, cinnamon, vanilla, and Lakanto. I warm everything up on a low flame on the stove top and add shredded coconut, raw nuts, etc. Then I refrigerate in small cupcake paper shells. Mmmmm, good!

When I want ice cream, I make coconut milk ice cream, Paleolithic style ice cream, or raw milk ice cream. Sometimes I make egg based ice cream, coined "get some" ice cream because it makes us ready for an intimate experience with our significant other. This was created by Dave Asprey of the Bulletproof Executive website. There are lots of varieties of non-junky ice cream recipes out there.

I know that we can enjoy all healthful, all delicious alternatives to what the mainstream dessert manufacturers offer to us. I find so many options these days that do not include sugar or grains. Every day it becomes easier and easier to just say no to conventional desserts. Challenge yourself! What's to lose, except illness, addiction, and bad habits?

FERMENTED FOODS

Naturally fermented foods are good for our intestines. They provide friendly bacteria which aid in digestion and keep the lining of our intestines healthy and functioning well. The good bacteria in naturally fermented foods are called probiotics. Some examples of these foods are raw organic sauerkraut, raw pickles, raw vinegar, plain yogurt from any animal, unpasteurized kefir or unpasteurized cheeses, unpasteurized sprouted miso, natto (fermented sprouted soy bean), kimchi, and kombucha tea.

Long term, these healthy bacteria can heal the gut and boost immunity. Some of the fermented foods mentioned here have an acquired taste. Some of these foods take a long time to make the correct way. Read the labels of store bought fermented foods, as added sugars and preservatives speed up the time from manufacturer to shelf, and this can negate any good the product may do. I love plain Greek yogurt and raw cheeses. I adore apple cider vinegar and balsamic vinegar. I add fermented foods to almost every meal. The stinky items (natto, miso), I use on occasion and definitely some time passed before my taste buds became accustomed to the unusual odors and flavors!

PROTEIN

Proteins have been mentioned already in other areas of this book. Proteins are tied into fats and probiotics, depending upon where they are sourced from.

Protein primarily feeds the muscle tissue, aids in repair and growth of the muscle tissue, and assists in the body's physical performance. When the protein leaves the stomach, it has been broken down into amino acids and carries oxygen throughout the body. We rely on food for our six essential amino acids. Those are the ones our bodies cannot manufacture on its own. Our bodies do have the capabilities to produce other amino acids without getting them from food.

It takes longer for the body to break down protein than sugars or carbohydrates, so protein keeps us fuller for a longer period of time. Protein uses up more energy in the digestion process too. Therefore, we burn more calories just by eating protein calories! Fat, however, keeps us fuller the longest of the three macronutrients; fat, carbohydrates, and sugar.

I like more bang for my buck, so to speak. I like the most protein grams per portion of food. If it is a low fat option of a high protein source, I feel free to add a healthy fat to the meal.

My favorite sources of whole food protein are wild caught fish and seafood, alligator, pastured chicken, and pastured eggs. My favorite supplemental foods for protein are raw dairy foods, Quest protein bars, organic gelatin powder, plain, nonfat Greek yogurt, 100 % egg protein powder, Pure Protein brand (35 gram) vanilla shake, raw nuts, seeds, and coconut.

I don't include beans in my diet because they take a lot of soaking and preparing for us to be able to digest them properly. They have way too much gas producing properties for me, and the carbohydrate load is way higher than the well advertised protein portion of beans. Then we have to look at the bioavailability of the human body to absorb the protein from beans. Some are better than others, but the body is trying to reject the bean in some way in order to cause such digestive distress (gas, bloating, diarrhea, etc.).

Notice the division between whole food proteins and supplemental proteins. One group is perfect for on-the-go days, and the other takes care and preparation. Of course the leftovers become the next day's on-the-run, grab-and-go food! It is a combination of the proteins, fats, vegetables, and fruits that work in beautiful symbiosis creating optimum health. Also note that some foods overlap into more than one nutrient area. A superior health leads to superior self, in more ways than one. Your radiant energy will emerge, and others will benefit from that energy. It is inevitable. The math with love and energy doesn't always make common sense. The more love and energy I feel, the more love and energy I have to give. And when I give it away, there's no subtraction of love and energy. I just keep gaining more! You will too.

LET'S TALK ABOUT SOY, BABY!

There has been a lot of information in the media about soy in recent years. Some paint it as a pretty picture, a vegan's protein dream. There is a health "halo" surrounding soy. Others look at soy as the body's own personal nightmare. Let's first dig into a little bit of the history of soy in the human diet, and then move into the nutritional profile of it, both pros and cons.

The soy bean crop originally was used thousands of years ago in Asia as a top crop, like fertilizer. It helped other crops grow because it fixed nitrogen in other crops and assisted in the absorption of oxygen.

Soy beans and their products were not even eaten by humans until 2500 years ago. The first form of soy being eaten was fermented soy made into a kind of paste, similar to our modern day miso. The miso paste and salt was utilized to preserve meats longer (as there was no refrigeration in those times). It was also added to soups.

In ancient China, monks were given tofu because it reduced their desire for sex. The testosterone hormone levels in the monks reduced and they could focus on their ritual duties much better. The tofu and soy products kept them, for the most part, honoring their vow of celibacy. In addition, the estrogen levels of the monks were elevated.

Nowadays the United States of America is the largest grower and exporter of soy in the world. Unfortunately, most of it is genetically modified and the seeds are owned by the giant company Monsanto.

Soy beans contain anti-nutrients, which are harmful to humans. In order for them to be non-damaging to us, they must be fermented or soaked. The soy products in our supermarkets are not as healthy as once thought. Soy is found in almost every packaged processed food. Personally, I can only find one brand of organic, wild sprouted, non GMO tofu in my grocery store. After reading and researching the truth about the hormone levels that can be altered by soy, I eat it sparingly.

In all of the products that the incredible edible soy is made into, it still is not a high source of protein. It is only about 61 percent protein and not all of that is bioavailable to the body. The rest of the nutrient makeup are carbohydrates and fat.

Basically, soy products are highly processed foods. It takes a lot to make soy milk and oil palatable. We don't find any soy products in nature, like a fruit, vegetable, flower, or animal.

CHOICES

Now that I have shared with you some truths about what I eat and what I don't eat, the choices are up to you. Healthy bodies look great by hard work *and* by accident. It takes moment-to-moment, smart choices that feed the inside, while the side effect is looking good on the outside. We are the byproduct of what we are doing daily in order to have optimum health.

Health is extremely personal and individual. Your body responds differently to what you put into it when compared to somebody else. There is a general consensus, however, that if we eat green leafy foods, pastured proteins, and good fats, our body will respond favorably when contrasted with when we eat junk food. That being said, tune into your instincts and primal intuition about what works for *you* in order to wake up each day with vitality. Now is the time to be selfish with your personal desires, research, and experimentation in order to reach towards your superior self.

Chapter Five

REACHING WAAAAY BACK TO THE FUTURE

*I*f we reach back far enough in human history, we find that human beings only began eating grains about ten thousand years ago, with the onset of the agricultural revolution. The population did not eat grains every day either, just like they didn't eat fruit every day. They ate these things when they were available, when they grew in their area under ideal climate conditions, and when they were ripe enough to fall or be picked without too much effort. In grains' case, they had to learn to soak and then grind them, before cooking over a fire. Only then, the grain was edible. Eating in a modern world with the principles of those who ate millions of years before grain was discovered and consumed is called many things. Some call it Paleolithic eating. Others refer to it as Primal eating. I have heard it named the Ancestral diet, the Evolutionary diet, and so on.

Fundamentally, if we eat as our forefathers did for millions of years before grains were consumed, we can see great improvements upon the Standard American Diet. Then we can see marked improvements in whole person care, not sick care. Taking the responsibility into our own hands instead of relying on doctors and pills to "fix" us is a large and empowering task. We are up to the challenge if we have the correct information and tools.

Many times when I am coaching people or when I am at the grocery store helping people learn how to shop to nourish the whole person, they will reach for the same edible food-like products they have put into their baskets for years. My eyebrows go up, my eyes widen in question, and this is usually the response given to me: "It's low fat, it's whole wheat, it's got vitamins and minerals added, it has the American Heart Association logo stamped on it!" My favorite answer is, "It's not for me, it's for the kids..."

You are not married to your past! Those past choices are what brought us to this disarrayed state of health in the first place. I am not saying that we are *bad* or guilty of wrong-doing. I'm saying that we have unfortunately been fooled for a long time by the mainstream food manufacturers and media dollars. Now we can choose differently. Now we have scientific research and success stories of friends and loved ones to provide both proof and anecdotal evidence that clean and green foods are the way to go. Create a new story.

Do I want my children to suffer the ups and downs of body weight and fat gain? Do I want my children to ride the emotional roller coaster of health drama and body image issues? No! So many of us have to come to this point in our lives where we have psychological damage caused by weight gain, as well as the mental and physical stress the accompanying chronic conditions create. I say it is time to think differently about body image. Create a new story for yourself and the generations to follow.

I encourage you to reach waaaay back to our ancient people's way of eating to ensure a brighter food and health future. Now is the time to go back to the beginning. We already have many convenience foods that are healthy for us when we are on the run. If you don't have time to cook or clean your foods properly, there is available ready-washed-and-cut greens and fruits at the grocery stores. Single serve packets of raw nuts and seeds are available for reasonable prices. The dollar store has so many fish and seafood canned in its own water, brine, or mustard with pop-tops. Read your labels carefully though. Use the modern conveniences without sacrificing your principles of health values and time values. It *is* doable. You got this!

When I began eating this way, I didn't even know there was a movement with a host of highly educated doctors, scientists, and fitness professionals working on sharing this information with the masses. I stumbled upon the data and the movement naturally as a result of the HCG protocol. Dr. Simeons did not call his approach to fat loss "Paleo," but it was. Habits take about 21 days to form. Dr. Simeons' protocol was about three weeks for the shortest round and about six weeks for the longest round. I feel that this was no mistake on his part. It was a brilliant plan. It was not a casual plan. Then, following the low calorie portion of the HCG protocol, one continues to eat more and more food choices, but absolutely no starches or sugars are eaten. Healthy fats are highly encouraged back into the diet. This perfectly sets us up for long term successful eating of live, healthy, real foods. It just so happens to be called "Paleo" in recent years.

The ground rules for the ancestral way of eating is to consume 100% pastured meats and eggs, fresh, wild caught fish and seafood, loads of non-starchy vegetables, fruits, nuts, and seeds on occasion. We are guided to steer away from beans, grains, dairy, added sugars, and processed junk foods.

It sounds simple, but it may not be easy. Being patient with ourselves is paramount. Dietary errors are normal during any new change in eating. When we acknowledge the error and do not dwell there, we can learn from it. Move on, move forward, and think about the good things you have done for your body thus far. These efforts to let go will work for any lifestyle changes or goals we want to accomplish. I say, "Shake that monkey off my back!"

If we eat in a Primal manner and tailor it to our specific likes and dislikes, coupled with paying attention to specific medical conditions, we can reduce or resolve many metabolic related disorders. Vegetables and most fruits are alkaline producing in the body, thus reducing inflammation and bone loss from acids in our systems. Proteins and fats take longer to digest, and burn more calories in the process of digesting, therefore we may feel fuller for a longer period of time when consuming them. We may consume less food but feel satisfied, especially if it is nutrient rich food. Fats also provide sharp mental focusing ability. The ancient ways of consuming food can improve our metabolism, and may improve insulin sensitivity.

Perhaps this information is great to hear and easy to understand, but putting it all into practical use for you and your family is a little overwhelming. Don't worry! I suggest in this case take baby steps. Baby steps are less intimidating for some folks. Inner strength helps us to chip away bit by bit at the changes we want to see inside our bodies and outside our bodies. Chipping away bit by bit towards our goals gives us more strength. So we see here the catch 22. When we are mentally strong, we feel empowered to make the small shifts that will in turn make us stronger! (What came first, the chicken or the egg?) A master marble sculptor still had to begin his masterpiece by chipping away bit by bit at the rough, not so perfect marble. In this case, you are the sculptor *and* the masterpiece!

Make a slight shift in your dietary approach with 100% commitment for one week. Each week add a new element to the already established changes. If one change a week is still too scary, make one change a month. I call them monthly promises instead of resolutions. We all made resolutions at the beginning of the year, every year, and by February they were abandoned. This may be more doable for you.

SUPERIOR SELF'S GUIDE TO
WELLNESS FROM WITHIN

The plan for you is week by week (or month by month).

I suggest:

Week 1, increase water to a gallon a day.

Here's why: Water consumption lubricates our entire body from the inside. It makes my joints less achy and my skin supple and fresh looking. Water assists in my digestive system moving food and their nutrients through my body and I am not constipated.

Fat cells may increase or decrease in size but we still have the same number of fat cells in our body since we were little (unless we surgically remove them). When we change our food intake to healthier choices, our fat cells may very well shrink. The fat that has been released needs to leave the body. Water consumption helps move the fat into elimination through our urine and sweat. The more water that goes in, the more water goes out. We also detoxify the body when we drink more water. When we drink lots of water, we may find ourselves satisfied with less food and our impulses to cheat fade away. I add yummy fresh flavors to pitchers of water in order to reach my goal of a gallon of water daily. I put sliced strawberries and mint leaves in one pitcher, sliced tomatoes and basil leaves in one pitcher, sliced cucumbers and cantaloupe in one pitcher, and lemon, lime, and orange slices in one pitcher. Sometimes I have to negotiate with my children concerning who gets the last glass of water!

Week 2, give up all wheat products, and still drink a gallon of water a day.

Here's why: Wheat and gluten are high on the food list that people are highly sensitive to in our world. Wheat and gluten containing products are in highly processed foods. Most commercial salad dressings have wheat and gluten in them, as well as a host of scientific sounding flavors and additives. Wheat and gluten act like glue in the body and make things "stick to our ribs." Wheat is one of the highest crops used in GMO farming practices. Wheat can be inflammatory in the body's systems. Most people are sensitive to wheat, but don't realize it. Yet when they follow my guide and give it up, they find aches, pains, gas, and bloating fading away.

Week 3, give up all grains, and still drink a gallon of water a day.

Here's why: All grains have to be processed in order to be edible. Those wheat berries, corn, millet, rye, barley, or oats must be picked, dried, split open, or ground. Then we must cook them in order to digest them. The smaller and finer the grind, the higher the glycemic index too. Extra fine bakers' flour has a much higher glycemic index than a wheat berry in its original form even though it is the same wheat. This spikes the insulin when ingested. The high energy spike is followed by a crash, and then low energy ensues. So we may reach for another high carbohydrate snack to raise our blood sugar levels again.

Week 4, reduce fruits to 1-2 times a day, always keeping previous changes.

Here's why: Fruits these days are sweeter than the ancient wild ones grown without agricultural practices. Thousands of years ago, fruit was eaten when in season and ripe. Our ancestors did not get to eat fruit very often. Today's fruit growers have perfected the colors and sizes to be uniform. As mentioned earlier, they are also grown sweet on purpose. This causes insulin spikes and cravings for more sweet tasting things.

Week 5, reduce fruits to 1-2 servings a week.

Here's why: Once we are able to conquer the fruit reduction to 1-2 times a day, it is time to lessen our fruit intake even more. I suggest substituting them with carrots, fennel, sweet potatoes, sweet peppers, winter squash, and raw chocolate! Reach for high fat foods instead of high sugar foods. This will keep our blood sugar levels more even throughout the day. You may find yourself not wanting fruits or sweet vegetables very often, after curtailing sweet produce consumption for a few weeks.

Week 6, change your oils to only healthy fats I mentioned earlier in Chapter 4.

Here's why: Fats and oils from minimally processed foods will provide energy for hours and a super satisfying, creamy mouth feel. My favorite afternoon pick-me-up is raw butter, raw milk cheese, and homemade, sugar-free preserves on a grain-free flax cracker. The high Omega 3 oils and lots of healthy fats will provide mental focus and clarity.

Week 7, no more added sugar, in any form: no honey or agave or date sugar. Buy Lakanto or XYLA on line or at health food stores.

Here's why: Some sugar substitutes that are sweet and natural still make our brains and bodies think we have had sugar. This triggers cravings. Remember that sweets are treats, not to be indulged in daily, even if it is natural.

Week 8, purchase raw dairy and pastured eggs if you regularly consume them.

Here's why: Raw dairy and 100% pastured eggs do not cause the same reaction to the body as grain fed animals. If sensitive to dairy and grains, one may not feel the reactions like with the grain fed products. My own experience is that I no longer suffer from constipation or rashes when I eat raw milk, cream, and cheeses. The pastured eggs just taste better, although I never had sensitivity to eggs.

Week 9, give up beans and legumes.

Here's why: Beans and legumes are high starch and must be soaked overnight and then cooked to release the gaseous property. For years the media has promoted beans as high protein, but most beans and legumes have about 30% protein. They must be processed for a long time in order to be bioavailable to the body. I tend to steer clear of them for my tummy's sake.

Week 10, write to me and share your experience!

I know you can do this. I want to hear from you so that I may better serve your needs. I want to know what was easier and what was more difficult to transition into. I want to know your triggers that usually cause you to give in to temptation, and if you became stronger than the cravings over time.

superiorselfwithkjlandis.com
Superior Self with KJ Landis on Facebook
kjlinsf@hotmail.com

In all of the weeks (or months), pay particular attention to how you feel rather than how you look. Sometimes flu and cold symptoms, headaches, and general fatigue may plague you. You may suffer acne or a rash for a little while. These are symptoms of the body detoxifying as it gets used to the cleaner fuel you are providing it with. Fear not, and keep moving forward with the process. Moving toward superior health can spur us on to our true superior self. Just think about how clear, attentive, helpful, and generous we can be to others we love after we have taken care of our own essential biochemical needs.

Practice, practice, practice. Eventually your eating choices and preparation of meals will shift to a healthier format and it will become easier. For me, it has not yet become entirely easy. It requires being present and conscious at each meal. Remember that you do not have to feel alone. Surround yourself with like minded individuals. Seek out thought provoking materials which stimulate your journey and continue to spark interest in your superior self.

Contemporary health and nutrition advice usually cycles through repetitions. We reach back to the adages of our ancestors. What is old becomes new again, for a time. The wave of the future came from waves of the past. Some habits stick with us and some don't. Our elders told us to eat our vegetables, go out and play, and get some rest. These words of wisdom ring true for me today. How about you?

I LIKE TO MOVE IT, MOVE IT!

Traditional exercise programs of the past fifty years varied immensely. Some schools of thought were focused on long bouts of cardiovascular exercise. Other programs were geared toward weight training only. Women were traditionally advised to do "aerobics" and "calisthenics." If we go waaaaay back, exercise was more functional. We gardened, hunted, gathered, walked, and played. We squatted while cooking and cleaning. We moved heavy things and sprinted when being chased or chasing something. These types of activities used more than one body part at a time. Survival was a workout in itself!

The current trend is to go back to functional movement exercise in order to live to a ripe old age without aches and pains. High intensity interval training uses bursts of speed and strength followed by moderate exertion or a short period of rest. It is very useful, efficient, and takes less time than chronic cardio or hours in the gym. Some examples of this are cross fit training, TRX training, capoeira, sprints followed by walking, etc. There are many opportunities to explore the so-called "new" workouts on the internet. See what appeals to you, and go for it! You have nothing to lose and everything good to gain. If you try some new exercise program and it turns out not to be fun for you, I suggest that you try something different. The key word is FUN! If something feels fun, there is a higher motivation to stick with it. If you see results in your body image, or results are progressing in your strength and stamina, this is all positive reinforcement of your health getting better and better. That can be extremely motivating to us, and we will probably go back to that activity go back one more time (or more).

When considering the types of movement that hunter-gatherers participated in, we must acknowledge that they had calm times of sitting around their shelters, stretching or working on weaving, skinning animals, and doing domestic type activities. They also foraged for food by walking hours a day.

In today's world, we have replaced walking all day looking for food with creating extra busy lives. We keep moving by over scheduling. We drive to most activities and usually sit at each event. Most desk jobs are done sitting. We look for *things to do* instead of looking for food. We look for money, relationships, clearances, clubs, and hobbies. Usually this disappoints us, so we keep moving on to other things to keep us busy. If we change this business of *busyness*, eat nourishing foods, and move around more, we can be happy with a less packed schedule.

YOGA

An ancient art of movement that is not quite as old as caveman activities, but still valuable for the body, mind, and spirit, is yoga. I am a huge fan of yoga, especially hot yoga.

Yoga practices go back more than 5000 years. It originated in India. The word *yoga* means to join together the mind and the body. It naturally incorporates breathing, exercise, and meditation. There are thousands of poses that we hold for a short time in order to strengthen the muscles and stretch them as well. Then we release the hold in order to replenish the muscles with a flush of fresh oxygen through the blood flow. The slow conscious breathing assists in holding the poses, we close our eyes in between poses, and at the end of class we are free to drift off into meditation or sleep. Some folks even say they leave their bodies for a few seconds! Sometimes yoga is called a moving meditation because some poses are so hard to do. For me, some poses I can only muster up the strength for a few seconds and I completely lose my mind. I can't think of anything, and when I lose my mind because it is so difficult, it *is* a kind of meditation. I think you do not have to be flexible to do yoga, but doing yoga will make you more flexible. It helps in the ease of other physical activities. It made me more flexible in the mind too. I get many of my brightest ideas during yoga class.

My favorite type of yoga is Bikram Hot Yoga. It is my latest obsession. Hot yoga is a guided 90 minute class in a room that is heated to 105 degrees fahrenheit. There are 26 poses repeated twice and two breathing exercises. I sweat profusely during class, and usually drink my mandatory one gallon a day of water during hot yoga.

My first class went something like this: I walked into the studio and it was eerily quiet. I thought it was an exercise class, not a meditation center! Then I went into the yoga room itself. I almost passed out from the stinky smell of sweaty feet and socks. There are no shoes or socks allowed in the area where yoga was practiced, so I knew it came from the buckets of sweat pouring off of the people practicing. Maybe it was the carpet absorbing the funk for years. When I asked about the odor, the staff said they steam cleaned the carpet daily. It is part of the culture of the environment, I guess. The room was damn hot too. The more people that showed up, the higher the room temperature got. It got up past 112 degrees.

I loved the fact that I was finally warm all over, from the inside out, from my bones to my skin! (After losing my chunk of weight, I was cold so often that I bought the biggest, baddest electric blanket I could find.) The class was hard and I perspired more than I had ever done before, even more sweat dripping off of me than when I ran a marathon! Then, after my first class, I needed a nap.

Something clicked in me. A new challenge! I was not going to let the stink and exhaustion win. I went back a few times that week. After about three weeks the odor magically didn't exist in my senses anymore, and exhaustion transformed into exhilaration. I am excited each night now to prepare my yoga bag for the next morning. On occasion, when I sleep only a few hours a night due to scheduling challenges, it is a complete deep sleep, and it leaves me satisfied and ready for more yoga.

The poses are meant for beginners. Every class is vocally instructed in the exact same way. It is up to practitioner to decide how far to push themselves. One gets more advanced by pushing deeper into the poses. Muscles are held tightly and blood flow is constricted, followed by release, and then fresh oxygenated blood travels rapidly to that area of the body. This is a high intensity cardio workout as well because when we grip with all of our God given power to our maximum capacity, the heart rate goes way up.

Stomach, stomach, stomach. The teachers emphasize tightening the abdomen throughout almost every pose to protect the lower back. This is beneficial to my body image and self esteem as well because the results are fabulous looking abdominal muscles. Strong abdominal muscles support the back muscles. I have recently seen tiny bulges of muscle in between my larger muscles, all over my body. (I have muscles. Even my muscles have muscles!) Hot yoga definitely supports the parts of our physique that some sports and exercise routines overlook. I'm nearly a half century old and I am as flexible as I was when I was in my late teens. Hot yoga never gets easier either! Every class is different depending upon my food and water intake, my mood, my quality of sleep, my work effort, etc. I keep waiting for it to become a breeze, yet it never does.

Some things I have noticed after more than a year of hot yoga are: my sweat does not sting my eyes anymore, I rarely catch a cold or flu, I heal rather rapidly from cuts and bruises, my menstruation does not provide me with mood swings, and I have a complete, restful sleep. I wake up thoroughly refreshed and ready to take on the day.

Hot yoga is a part of my regime, but not my complete routine. It prepares me for jogging, spinning, weight training, hiking, and serving food and beverages as a server for six to eight hours in the evenings.

I heartily encourage everybody to search and experiment with many forms of physical movement. See what makes you happy for any amount of time each day. A happy exerciser will spill some of that happiness onto someone else. That contagious energy is a gift to somebody who may have just needed a jolt of love at that very moment. If you are not a loner by nature (and we humans are social creatures...), enlist others to join you. There is power in numbers and a sense of accountability too. Making plans with somebody else on their road to health and fitness may just push you to suit up and show up. That is one step closer to your superior self.

STONE AGE AND MODERN CLANS

The human survival and ability to thrive has always depended upon being with others. The cave man hunted in groups while his mate and children gathered food and supplies. The primitive cultures included community and social connections, even if it was only a few people gathering or living together. Sharing meals, tasks, and stories assisted the human race in growing and developing vigorously.

Our modern clans, that is, our families, work families, religious and school families, hobby and club families, and circle of friends are what keep us feeling connected to each other and to our higher power. This is what I believe. We call upon their strengths and aid when we feel like we just can't do this life thing, this diet thing, this challenge of this very moment, all by ourselves.

During our initial efforts of changing to an optimal nutrition lifestyle, it is important to establish a support system. Find someone who looks the way you want to look, who exudes buckets of joy, positive energy, and grace. Ask them what they are eating, drinking, and what physical activities they do to stay fit! People love to be admired for the things they are doing well, and honest compliments open up a heart dialogue. Your spouse or partner may be ready to go on this journey alongside of you. Taking the children, elders, cousins, or aforementioned types of family members along the path with you may be just what is needed to impact *all* of your tribe toward a flourishing life.

We need allies to put up a united front against the health misconceptions and misinformation of the past 80 years. We need allies to put up a united front against cravings, poor food choices, and impulsive food shopping. "No man is an island, no man stands alone." Joan Baez wrote this song years ago and the message rings true today. The cliché of old habits dying hard is equally true. It is an everyday thing, this health journey. I'm not suffering by any means when I choose foods that enrich my biology, but it is a mental piece of work that is carried out *every single time.* I would rather carry the work out with my tribe at my side.

Nobody is 100% perfect on any protocol 100% of the time. There has to be a level of self forgiveness and a level of forgiveness towards others in your community. We have the opportunity to be non-judgmental at the same time that we are striving for growth and vitality. If one is committed and has a long term vision, eventually the desired results will appear.

With your tribe backing you up, your goal setting can go a little wild! Some of the most supportive people I have met while on my journey to my superior self have been complete strangers in real life. They have been on discussion forums and social media on the internet. Perhaps because they don't live with me or see me daily, they can give 100% to being my champion and hold me accountable to my seemingly outrageous personal goals. What little time they do give to me is very much focused and present. I am forever grateful and humbled by the experience. Be fearless in assembling your own clan. Each small step taken in the direction of your goals is an invisible pat on the back. Just do it, and see what wonderful things come your way!

Chapter Six

ALTERNATIVE CANCER AND HEALING THERAPIES

*W*e human beings are exceedingly stubborn. We have to be in extreme pain, scared out of our wits, or desperate beyond compare in order to do the work that we need to do to heal ourselves. When we let go of our limited thinking, real change can occur.

During the past couple of years I have been keenly interested in how the HCG protocol, the whole foods eating style, and the Paleo/Primal way of eating can assist in the healing of obesity related medical conditions. The foods eaten during the HCG protocol are clean and green, nutrient rich, and high in protein. The same goes for the other real food protocols. As I researched alternative healing therapies with food based medicines, I came across four natural therapies that were similar in food content to the HCG protocol. They were used successfully in treating cancer and other chronic conditions.

For many years the mainstream cancer industry and cancer research industry has focused mainly on the cancer cells themselves. Kill the cancer cells without any regard to the whole human being. I am certain that you, the reader, have known somebody with cancer, and have seen the decline in their health through chemotherapy and radiation. I have, and it is not very pretty. I believe that we should be focusing on whole person care and preventive care.

Our modern system of health care can save time, money, and lives when we pay attention to whole person care, optimum healing through our food intake, and prevention of illness. We can be vital and active our whole lives if we take steps to ensure that happens. I want to be fully functioning at 90 or more, and die peacefully in my sleep when my time comes to leave this planet.

These four alternative healing therapies rely on the environment in the entire human body where the cancer cells live and thrive. If we can significantly change the environment where cancer cells reside, the cancer cells can no longer survive and multiply. The four therapies that have intrigued me the most are:

- **The Gerson Therapy**
- **The Budwig Diet**
- **The Burzynski Antineoplaston Treatment**
- **Dr. Simoncini's Sodium Bicarbonate Therapy**

The Gerson Therapy

Dr. Max Gerson wrote a book in 1958 that covered thirty years of his remarkable work with cancer patients. One of his fundamental beliefs was that the soil was our external metabolism and that if we take care of the soil, the things that we receive from the soil will take care of us in the long term. He was an environmentalist of sorts. Treating our bodies with foods that came from untainted soil is the basis of what we now call organic gardening. Dr. Max Gerson practiced what Hippocrates said so famously, "Let food be thy medicine and medicine be thy food."

Dr. Gerson's therapy worked equally well on acute and degenerative diseases. One of his most well known patients was Dr. Albert Schweitzer. The Gerson Therapy cured Schweitzer's adult onset diabetes. What's even more shocking to know is that it was completely reversed in six weeks! Dr. Gerson's methods were considered controversial in the first half of the 20th century because he was treating formerly incurable diseases with diet. This type of therapy didn't take care of American economics at the time. The United States was just getting into new fangled, processed, packaged convenience foods. The stock market was paying attention to the new foods and vegetable oils that were emerging in the food industry.

The Gerson Therapy took care of people first, and placed humanity above industry. That is one of the reasons why the information is not plastered across billboards, posters, and brochures nationwide. It was thrown under the rug in the senate of the U.S. when a bill Dr. Gerson wrote got lots of attention. His bill, named the Pepper-Neely Anti-Cancer bill was shared with doctors who were also senators. There was a consensus among them that natural healing of cancer would dampen the American economy.

His daughter Charlotte Gerson, who is now in her early nineties, still carries on her father's work at The Gerson Institute, with centers near San Diego and in Mexico.

The basic nutritional concept of the Gerson Therapy is that we flood the ill person with nutrient dense foods that bring the whole body back to optimum health. What this entails is ingesting lots of raw vegetable juices made fresh, three times a day. This gives a large amount of oxygen and live enzymes to every cell, which therefore promote healing. Organic, raw, and cooked produce are also permitted. For the first few months there is no meat and very little salt taken. Very little fats are included. One oil that is permitted is cold pressed flax seed oil. It has a high concentration of Omega 3 fatty acids. Dr. Gerson found that these fatty acids can kill human cancer cells without killing normal cells.

After the initial few months, organic, 100% pastured meats, eggs, and wild caught fish are permitted. Nonfat Greek yogurt and cottage cheese may be added eventually.

Dr. Gerson observed that this type of eating speeds up the cell turnover and increases metabolism.

Raw, organic apple cider vinegar is encouraged. It tastes acidic but promotes alkalinity and good bacteria in the body. The food choices permitted in healing the cancer cells are so similar to the clean eating protocol of the HCG protocol. I compared the two and saw the healing properties of both diets. When we promote an alkaline environment in the body and add super nutrition, cancer cells cannot grow. In the Gerson Therapy some patients have received full remission.

The Gerson Therapy also employs the use of organic coffee enemas several times a day. This encourages a detoxification of the body, especially the liver. Patients tell of an immediate relief of aches and pains caused by the cancer.

The Gerson Therapy is preventive in many diseases and builds up the immune system through nutritional intake. The HCG protocol and my further quest of extreme clean eating have done the same for me. I am extremely healthy, active, and full of positive energy, now that I have a nutrient dense food intake. I haven't had a cold or flu for a very long time.

More information is freely available on the internet on Gersonmedia.com and Gersoninstitute.org. There are resources at your local library as well.

The Budwig Diet

The Budwig Diet has been called an anti-cancer diet as well. Like The Gerson Therapy, it too has been helping successfully with arthritis, blood pressure problems, diabetes, fibromyalgia, psoriasis, eczema, and cancer.

Dr. Johanna Budwig was a seven time Nobel Prize nominee in the 20th century for her work with helping fight cancer in its most hopeless cases. Dr. Budwig believed that all states of illness or health begins in the gut. The Standard American Diet of highly processed and refined foods, the use of vegetable oils, and toxic dirt creates an imbalanced chemistry in the body. This is called a lack of homeostasis.

This lack causes the body to have less energy and less electricity, similar to a lower watt light bulb versus a higher watt light bulb. This lower energy can cause a poor circulation and systemic problems, with less oxygen reaching every cell. Dr. Budwig's therapy was similar to Dr. Gerson in that she treated cancer patients with high amounts of vegetable juices. She believed that the super concentrated nutrients from these juices were essential for healing.

In her work, Dr. Budwig discovered that when she combined cold pressed, organic, raw flax seed oil with cottage cheese or quark (a type of European cottage cheese), the chemical reaction from the combination of foods made the oils and water more easily absorbed into the cells. The essential fatty acids in this combination of cottage cheese and flax seed oil also helped other nutrients to be absorbed. Changing the internal environment of our body is essential to making a place where cancer cannot thrive, or even survive. Dr. Budwig worked on the premise that cancer was a result of the problem. The problem seemed to be that a person was unhealthy in their diet and lifestyle. She did not believe that cancer was the cause of the problem.

Both Dr. Budwig and Dr. Gerson believed that cancer could not survive in an alkaline environment. Processed foods and sugars create an acidic environment where cancer can grow. My current eating style embraces foods that lower acidity and raise alkalinity in the body. Nutritional restoration, and changing habits to better our food choices are also the basis of the HCG protocol.

The Budwig Anti-Cancer Diet starts with a porridge-like substance of the flax seed oil and cottage cheese. This is made fresh three times a day. It is blended until smooth, like a ricotta cheese texture. One may add in raw nuts, cinnamon, cayenne, or fruits.

The rest of the diet includes raw nuts, raw seeds, and raw oils, especially coconut. It uses spices, herbs, raw fermented vegetables, raw vegetable and fruit juices, fresh fish, and 100% pastured eggs. No animal fats or hydrogenated oils are allowed. No high mercury shellfish is permitted. No soy, corn, or the many names for sugar are permitted.

This sounds familiar to me! The Budwig Diet recommends 80% raw foods and 20% cooked foods. This is right in line with the HCG Body for Life protocol. After Phase 4, I eat 80%-90% clean, whole, real foods and 10%-20% planned treats now and then.

Dr. Johanna Budwig encouraged the elimination of all toxic foods, all preservatives, additives, dyes, pesticides, artificial colors, and flavorings. She did permit flours if they were whole grain and organic. Johanna Budwig said, "If God made it, we can eat it, but try to eat it in the form that God made it."

I love that message!

Dr. Budwig noticed that many of her cancer patients had Candida infections. Candida is a fungal infection caused by the body not being able to oxygenate well. She found that if we feed the body with super nutrients we can eliminate fungal Candida, and rid the body of cancer. A grain free and sugar free diet will eliminate the Candida from the body. This type of diet will reduce inflammation as well, which adds to relief of pain and other symptoms of chronic conditions.

Dr. Budwig believed in massage and saunas to further remove toxins from the lymphatic system. The foods ingested combined with detoxification can renew the body's environment and heal cancer.

There is more information available for free at www. budwigcenter.com. There is a free download in PDF form and free references listed there as well.

Dr. Burzynski's Antineoplaston Treatment

Dr. Stanislav Burzynski created the term antineoplaston. What does it mean? Anti means against. Neoplaston is a cancer cell. In 1967 in his clinic, Dr. Burzynski discovered that a particular bond of two or more amino acids is naturally found in humans. These particular bonds are the body's natural biochemical defense system. People with cancer don't have enough of this naturally occurring antineoplastons within their body. Healthy people without cancer have plenty enough. These amino acid peptide bonds work independently of the regular immune system. They have the capability to turn off the genes that cause cancer.

Originally the antineoplastons were sourced from human blood and urine, but now they are synthetically made in Dr. Burzynski's laboratory. The treatment involves taking them by mouth or by injection, in the veins or muscles. These treatments may last eight months to a year.

The FDA has opposed the successful treatments because it is something that is found naturally in the body. It is not a huge moneymaker for the drug industry.

The similarities between the Burzynski Treatment and the HCG protocol are that both are found naturally in the body, both are taken orally or by injection, and both have been shunned by the FDA.

The diet on the Burzynski Treatment is very similar to the HCG protocol. Dr. Burzynski stated that we don't want to feed the cancer with refined carbohydrates and sugar. The clinic uses turmeric, garlic, onions, and curry powder daily in order to reduce inflammation in the body. Dr. Burzynski also claimed that exercise and vitamin D is important, and he believes the mind is a powerful tool in addressing diseases. Furthermore, Dr. Burzynski's clinic in Texas takes each patient on a nutritional protocol journey that is personalized just for them.

Similar to the HCG Body for Life Protocol, Dr. Burzynski recommends large amounts of water in order to flush out toxins and keep sodium levels down naturally.

There is no money to be made in finding a permanent cure for cancer. That is why it has not been done yet. In my opinion these underground therapies have just as much a chance to help heal without the toxic side effects that chemotherapy and radiation provide.

For more information and insight, please view the film called Burzynski: The Movie. It is free on YouTube.

Dr. Simoncini's Sodium Bicarbonate Therapy

Dr. Tullio Simoncini is an oncologist in Rome. He promotes treating cancer with sodium bicarbonate, which is essentially baking soda! His theory is that basically all cancers are a result of the presence of a fungus within the body. When cancer patients pass away and an autopsy is performed, a fungus is always present in the body, especially in the area of the tumors.

Dr. Simoncini has been using sodium bicarbonate for over twenty years in his clinic. Sodium bicarbonate is administered directly on the tumor. it can be used orally, in the arteries with an I.V., or injected into the tumor site. The sodium bicarbonate can penetrate any fungus in the body and the fungus does not become immune to it. It rapidly disintegrates tumors. If there are tumors in the vagina area, the area is douched with the sodium bicarbonate. If there is cancer in the lower colon or anus, the clinic uses enemas.

There are no side effects or after effects and the use of the sodium bicarbonate is fast, efficient, and inexpensive. The regression rate of the cancer is usually seen to begin within 45 days. Like the three other alternative cancer therapies, this treatment is used in other chronic illnesses also. Dr. Simoncini believes that if we eliminate the fungus we can eliminate the cancer (and other illnesses). The baking soda results in the alkalinization of the tumors and the area around the tumors.

The nutrition on the Simoncini treatment encourages foods that reduce acid in the body and increases alkalinity throughout the body. Foods that are alkaline and can be included in his treatment are again very similar to those used in the HCG protocol.

They are:

- asparagus
- onions

- vegetable juices
- parsley
- raw spinach
- broccoli
- garlic
- celery
- lettuce
- zucchini
- almonds
- flax seed oil
- stevia
- luo han gao (monkfruit)
- tomatoes
- mushrooms
- cabbage

Sounds a little familiar, no? To wrap it all up, the message I received from these four doctors of alternative healing therapies is: if we eat real foods, lots of leafy greens, things easily found in nature, we can prevent or cure many chronic illnesses, including cancer. I am not a doctor and I strongly suggest that you do your own research to thoroughly understand each of these therapies outlined here. Please consult with your health care practitioner before embarking upon any treatment for illness. Remember though...if eating poor processed food choices, laden with chemicals, artificial flavors, colors, and preservatives broke us, it would seem natural to turn to a non-chemical laden treatment to help fix us. Why pop a pill when we can reach for something immensely healthier and with the potential to heal without side effects?

The pharmaceutical industry is the single most profitable industry on the planet. Even if one does choose the conventional methods of cancer treatment in our modern society, the alternative treatments presented here can be used alongside or afterwards. The goal is to feel better inside and out. The journey of exactly how to do that is unique and personal to each individual.

Chapter Seven

SIMPLE VS EASY

With the information gathered so far from this book, it should come as no surprise that the lifestyles changes and particular protocols are relatively simple. Simple, however, is not equal to easy. Habits we have participated in for years and years are not easily broken. That's another reason why this book was written: to show you the optional ways to shift to a healthier lifestyle, and how they can overlap. Each formula is specific and each formula works if you follow it exactly as written. You cannot fail yourself if you at least implement one small change with 100% commitment once in a while. Then you move on to the next shift. That's the way permanent change occurs, bit by bit.

What diet or eating protocol is right for you? The diet that one can follow with consistency for a long time is the winner. It is divorcing the thought that the word diet equals short term lifestyle changes, and going without. It is changing the idea that diet is a lack of something, a void in what foods make us happy.

Food makes us happy? Where did that come from? Food is nourishment for the body so that the body can perform efficiently and with ease. Food is fuel so that our bodies can function well. Think about which of the protocols resonate with your body, spirit, heart, and lifestyle. Which one seems *doable*, regardless of the surrounding environment? Then as time goes on, and the brain is accustomed to the new food choices and habits, we can tweak and experiment without fear. Your body knows what to do if you trust it.

We humans have some sort of self evaluation going on all of the time. As we become comfortable with our new system of eating, we can evaluate our progress without judgment and then experiment accordingly. How do you feel? How are your blood tests and other health markers improving? Are you responding with strength, renewed energy, agility, better sleep, a sense of well being?

Notice that I didn't say *try*. Trying creates a state of trying again and again. Trying creates a test of some sort, with one foot in the circle and one foot out of the circle. Commitment requires *doing*.

We all have heard of "try before you buy." I'm not offering a TRY. I am offering a DO.

One evening a couple of years ago, my husband and I were on a date night. We were parked early for a jazz concert and were sitting and chatting in the car. He held a lip balm in the palm of his right hand. He asked me to try and take the lip balm from the palm of his hand. (I love games!) I reached over to grab it and quick as a flash he closed his fist. We played a few rounds of this game. "Come *ooonnnn*, do it!" he said vehemently. I kept saying, "I *am* trying!" I was frustrated but having fun at the same time. He smiled and looked at me quietly. Ooooh, point well taken. Exactly. Are you trying or are you doing? Trying led me to more trying. Doing may have led me to completing the task. Do you TRY or DO?

These protocols are simple, yet hard. Anything worth doing correctly the very first time takes grit. Anything worth doing correctly the one hundredth time takes grit! It takes a level of stepping out onto uncharted territory. Simple is not the same thing as easy. Complicated is not the same thing as hard.

Hard is climbing Mount Everest, but it is relatively simple. Place one foot in front of the other. Repeat. Repeat. Repeat. Eventually one will arrive at the top of Mount Everest. Hard is running a marathon. Place one foot in front of the other. Repeat. Repeat. Repeat. Simple rules to follow, but great effort and commitment entailed. Get my point?

The path to our superior self is a simple one: move lots, lift heavy things, play, laugh, eat food in the closest form that God made it, and pray a small prayer of gratefulness. This is not easy, but it is simple. Re-examine why you are reading this book and what brought you here in the first place. Streamline the distractions and focus on the bigger picture: YOU.

Old habits produce old results. New habits produce new results. Let nothing distract you from any goal. Let's break the word *nothing* down. It is *no* and *thing*. Let *no thing* distract you from your goal, even if it is your own ego in your head telling you that you can't, you aren't that special, you failed so many times before, etc...

Send negativity on its merry way. I write down negative thoughts on paper and tear them into thin strips. I roll the strips up into little scrolls, and burn them in a small clay flower pot outside. It feels so good to know that I physically acknowledge that the negative thoughts exist, and I can physically do something about it. *That* is tangible and satisfying to me. I call it my Negative Thought Pot. When I have burned up the negative thoughts, I allow space in my head and heart for something positive and different to enter my being. I know you all have an empty clay pot somewhere or you can get one at the dollar store. I did. Practice examining the negative thoughts that keep you stuck when you want to move forward. When you have a fear or inconsistency in your life, write it down and burn it up. It will empower you. I practice this with my kids and my coaching clients. Allowing possibilities to fly in from the universe can be pretty exciting. It sets the tone for new adventures to enter your life.

There are common threads running through these wellness protocols presented here. It is up to us to begin to feel better about our lives, mentally, physically, and spiritually. It takes a decision followed by an action. Choose to act rather than react. Reacting is allowing the ego and the negative talk to be around you again, and to rule you again. Let's break down the word *react*.

It is *re* and *act*. That means to act again, again, and again in the same expected way. That is what the ego does. It creates the same sad story and negative self talk that we are used to. We just burned those up and destroyed them, remember?

Choose wisely, and then stick with it until you have the goal in the palm of your hand. Whether it is weight loss, fat loss, weight gain, muscle building, pain relief, disease relief...see it through for the recommended allotment of time. Then, and only then, play around with your desires, as long as they fit in with the permanent lifestyle changes made without sabotaging the long term efforts. I freely have dark, sugar free, raw chocolate, and alcohol a couple of times a week after establishing my ground rules that worked for me. If I stick to my standards of clean eating 80 to 90 percent of the time, I do not gain weight or fat.

Each optimum lifestyle plan presented here has nutrient dense and very satisfying foods, as well as lots and lots of water. You will gain a renewal of the six senses. You will have an appreciation for who you are and what the universe has to offer you. I believe the universe will also supply you with worthwhile people who will support you, while all along showing you what abundant things you have to share with the world.

Once you are at the "feeling great" stage of your life, once you are bursting with energy, then a sense of play enters your arena. You can experiment with recipes, nutrient values in the diet, etc. I usually post meal photos and recipe ideas on my Facebook page and my website. They are meals truly thrown together. I don't measure ingredients very often, much to my mother's dismay. She has two bookcases full of cookbooks dating back more than a century. Using exact quantities in my meal planning takes the creative aspect away from me.

I believe the imagination is such a mind blowing and mind opening gift from God. Imagine yourself at the size and shape of your dreams. Imagine yourself free from aches and pains every day. Imagine yourself healing quickly and completely from routine headaches, rashes, and injuries. Imagine yourself having so much energy and power that you must give some away to feel whole! BONUS! Everybody gets a little piece of your heart.

The only way to get comfortable with doing something is to get uncomfortable for a while. My niece was hill training with me recently and she had never run up the very steep San Francisco hills that I chose for our challenge. We ran straight up hill, slowly, for about 25 minutes. Then we entered the wooded path at the very top. After 25 minutes of the steep hill training, the rest of the run had definitely taken on an easier feel.

After the run, we were guzzling water in my kitchen. I asked her the feelings she had about the experience. That's when she told me the only way to get comfortable with doing something is to get uncomfortable. She said that she knew it would become easier after repeated efforts, so she was committed to coming back and doing the hill regularly. She also stated that she had to make that kick-ass run her "bitch."

That's what a warrior does. Instead of giving the power to the hill, she used the power of the hard climb as motivation to not fear the hill, to own the hill, to accept the power it provides when coming to the top, and to realize just how far up we had journeyed. Anything can become comfortable, but first when we attempt it we must embrace getting uncomfortable. After eight years of running two miles straight up, up, up, that daunting hill has become a close friend of mine.

To me, the hill is a metaphor for any life challenges. It was simple. Put one foot in front of the other. Repeat. Repeat. Repeat. Simple, yes. Easy, no. Maybe you have challenges ahead that seem overwhelming or impossible. Maybe you are thinking to yourself that you can't run a mountain trail. Maybe you are thinking that you are too fat, too sick, too achy, too out of shape, too inexperienced. Perhaps your personal challenge will be to walk for five minutes on a level plane without intermission. Make the task at hand your ally, little by little. We were all beginners at *something* at *some* time! This is no different.

Choosing new foods, severing food addictions, learning alternative healing therapies, exercising with a different point of view, are all *doable*. Know it. Believe it. Baby steps will take you there. Make the time you spend with your food, your learning, and your exercise count. Treasure it as sacred because *you* are sacred. You deserve to be in a superior state of health. Become your superior self.

Chapter Eight

THAT'S THE WAY, "AH-HA, AH-HA" I LIKE IT!

*W*e all have *a-ha* moments throughout our lives, every day even, if we slow down long enough to acknowledge them. Igniting that spark of a deeper understanding of who we ultimately are may come from a book, a teacher, a friend, a family member, a poster on the side of a bus stop, a movie, a song, or a speech. Reaching down into our own hearts and into the hearts of others may come from something large or small, ordinary or extraordinary. The knock of the invisible hand on the door of knowledge, and appreciation of our existence does not discriminate. Are you awake to change? I am, now, but I wasn't always.

I was stubborn and closed minded to miracles for many years, even as they were happening right in front of me. I rationalized and gave excuses for the miracles, the coincidences. I placed everything into its little box, into its imaginary set of drawers in my organized mind.

Losing weight so rapidly without being ill raised not only my eyebrows, but everybody in my home, family, and work community was astounded. As I finished my journey of fat and weight loss, another journey of discovery began. I began vigorously researching cutting edge health and fitness information. Suddenly my spiritual awakening was rapidly expanding in tiny movements, daily. I found words of wisdom speaking directly to me from multiple sources all of the time. They were probably there all along, but now I was awake and ready to fully receive the gifts.

Here are some words of wisdom, stories, thoughts, and quotes bestowed upon me, and how they relate to the challenges of health and vitality. They spoke to me in other ways too, in my big life goals. My desire is that as you read this chapter you will develop a sense of awareness and sensitivity to the events happening around you daily. Think about how they can inspire and provide insight into you becoming the better version of you, for now. Then, tomorrow, you get to do it all over again! How lucky and blessed we are!

"Overlooking is better than not looking at all."
~Elton Thanh

Elton is a server with me at the restaurant where we work. We were busy one night, and as I was setting up a table for a large group, I overlooked a dirty glass. I thought I was perfectly prepared. Elton noticed the dirty glass and replaced it. I told him that I must have overlooked it. That's when he said the quote.

To me, this means that we humans do the best we can, we give our best preparation, and still we may overlook something and make a mistake. If I had never done the work in the first place, and was not lucky to have a partner who cared enough to help check that everything was in its place, we both would have missed it. His quote means he cared.

Care enough about your health goals to make a plan, a list, shop smart, and hold yourself responsible and accountable. Still, mistakes may be made, but far less than if you did not care. Elicit support, and seek checks and balances from those around you who also care deeply about your goals. More eyes on the prize...

"If I am not for myself, then
who is for me? And if I am only
for myself, then what am I?"
~Hillel

To me, this quote means toot your own horn! Be proud of every little step made in the direction of your goal. Don't be humble to the point of putting yourself down or belittling your accomplishments. It also means that we should spread the word, spread the love, and not be selfish with what we discover along the way. Spread your passions, and pay it forward.

"The waves, the waves,
occurring and occurring...
Threaten to drown me, until I realize
that I...am...the...ocean."
~Scott McInnes

This short poem came from my husband's college roommate. It describes how humans can get caught up and snagged in the little things, and we then disregard the bigger picture. Small errors in the healthy new protocol we have chosen may be disregarded because in the bigger picture, we are mostly there and moving forward. We are all particles of something bigger and unifying in nature.

"Even a broken clock gives the
correct time twice a day."
~Joe Rogan podcast

This hilarious quote is saying that even if something is bad, it has the capability to give something good and right some of the time. If I know the information someone is giving me is 100% wrong, but they are sharing from their heart, I can keep my mouth shut long enough to acknowledge their choice to give freely. I am grateful for that moment of connection.

"The path with heart does not
make you work at liking it."
~T. Von Jones

When something feels right there is a certain flow, with much less tension and rough spots. There is less grating on the nerves all of the time. When we fall in love with the right person for us right now, or when we eat in a healing manner now, it is easier to navigate through life, and it continues to get easier day by day. When you know, you *know*.

"Compassionate capitalism."
~Carl McCarden

There is a way to be a money maker in our world and still take care of people's hearts. There is a way to eat abundantly and enjoy treats without sabotaging your own greater good.

"Risk little, win little."
~KJ Landis

Don't cling to fear. Sometimes in life we must take a risk in order to grow. The rewards may be great or small, but we will never find out if we don't take chances.

"We are living life out of sequence."
~T. Von Jones

One warm evening in San Francisco, my husband and I were out to dinner. My husband ordered dessert first. I looked at him and exclaimed, "We are eating dinner out of sequence!" He had a wide grin on his face when he said that we were living life out of sequence.

To me, this means we can shake it up! We don't have to stick to the normal status quo in our daily lives. When we do something unexpected, no matter how small, it creates a rush of energy throughout our minds and bodies. Our heart rate increases, and we get happy! This also can help us see things from another person's point of view.

> "If you don't have the courage to say something,
> have the courage to leave the room."
> **~Maya Angelou**

Maya Angelou was a guest speaker at my church the day my son was baptized. She led the sermon that day. She was talking about racial and social justice. Some people just aren't comfortable with confrontation. Her message was that if something really is at odds with your soul and you can't speak up, then your statement will be heard loud and clear when you stand up and leave the room.

The same goes for our well meaning friends that sometimes attempt to sabotage our new healthy goals. Which is it, support or sabotage? They say they support us, but continue to bring chips, cakes, cookies, pies, fast foods, etc. to the office or to pot luck parties. On birthdays, they are the ones who bring sweets and alcohol even though they know you are on a different track now. "Just this once, you deserve it! You've been doing so well and look good now!"

My point exactly. If we aren't done with our weight loss journey yet and don't want to lecture the friends again and again, LEAVE THE ROOM. You will empower yourself by doing so. Do not let others dictate who you are. You know who you are and you know the road you are on.

"Let's reverse industry above humanity."
~T. Von Jones

Here is another winning quote from my prolific husband. As I learned more and more about the processed food industry and their ways of using GMOs, growth hormones, chemicals, sugars, addictive substances, and advertising in order to make us think their products are good for us, I would rant at the kitchen table. He listened (and still listens...it's in his contract!) to my enthusiastic goals, and said that I had a responsibility to the planet now that I was in the know. I was obligated to share the truth and dispel the myths. I was meant to expose the lies, and reverse the theme of industry above humanity. Thank you, honey.

"Guilt says I made a mistake.
Shame says I am a mistake."
~Dr. Christiane Northrup

When we eat off protocol of whatever plan we have chosen to embrace, we feel guilty. When we skip a day of movement or miss an exercise class we have signed up for, we are embarrassed. This is just a mistake. We can move forward from this and get over the guilt. We can forgive ourselves, and change our habit or choice the next time around. Shame, on the other hand, says we suck. We are worthless. Our value is diminished.

I am here to tell you that you are not a mistake. You have no place holder on the shame label. You are worthy of abundance, love, and light. You are a treasure. Ask those around you if you don't believe me! We all make errors on the winding and bumpy road that this life is. Stand back up. Carry on. The load does get lighter, and you will see clearer one day soon.

"A set back is a set up for a comeback."
~Pastor Douglass Fitch

I'm not sure if my pastor was the first one to say this, but he was the first person that shared this quote with me. When we have set backs in our health, our jobs, or our big plans, we get discouraged beyond belief. Instead, we can use the set back to regroup our ideas and plans. Take inventory of what is going on in your life that is going well, and be grateful for it. The lull in action may be just the pause needed before propelling into action once again. We will be stronger, do more good for ourselves, do more for others when we do spring back. Watch out!

"Who you are is not what you did."
~Taylor Swift

I was jogging one afternoon at the beach and this song called "Innocent" came on my iPod. This quote was in the song's chorus. The line spoke to me because humans do stupid things multiple times a day. We think stupid things multiple times a day. That does not mean we are our stupid thoughts or actions. We can own our beautiful spirits, claim our right to grow, and be special despite the silly things we say and do.

"There is only one purpose for all life, and that is for you and all that lives to experience fullest glory."
~Neal Donald Walsh

My favorite nonfiction book of all time is *CONVERSATIONS WITH GOD, Book 1*. The entire book forever changed how I view and reacted to people. Almost every page had mind blowing a-ha moments for me. This particular quote revealed that I can be the very best expression of myself. That is attainable not only to me, but to all human beings! Sometimes I am giddy with joy when I recall this. The good news is, you are invited to this party too!

> "Tremendous things are in store for you.
> Many wonderful surprises await you!"
> **~Willy Wonka character**

Every day we get the opportunity to learn a new thing or to see things from a new point of view. It is a gift. Each moment we have the chance to discover strengths we didn't even know existed or that we possessed. Invite surprises into your life.

> "Let freedom reign."
> **~Chrisette Michele**

On another jogging day, I listened to this song with open ears, mind, and heart. Oh, I get it. To me, this message says that we have the luck in this country to pretty much do whatever we like to do as long as we don't hurt anybody. Freedom is king, freedom rocks, freedom rules! Freedom does not always come so easily though. Like respect, it must be earned, and unfortunately, battles of the mind, body, and spirit are fought to reach that freedom spot. I also say let freedom *rain*. We have so many choices at our fingertips in the modern world. I am grateful for these freedoms that rain down upon me. This obesity thing, and the medical conditions that ride alongside of it, are "first world" problems, really. We are lucky to have so many choices, healthy or unhealthy! What an overwhelming blessing! Think about it!

My purpose and passion with the insights I received have not waned over time. I rise up each day eager to help, to heal, and to guide the planet towards real solutions to the problems in our lives. Never underestimate your drive or your power to do all of these things too. Once you get it, you *get it*.

Chapter Nine

FREQUENTLY ASKED QUESTIONS

*W*hen people hear about my body transformation and renewed quest for balance in mind, body, and spirit, I often get questions regarding their own pathways toward their health and wellness goals. When we reflect upon things that we did and knew they weren't life affirming, we have questions about how exactly to proceed differently. Here, I will share some frequently asked questions and my answers. It is my hope that the advice given here will assist you on the road to feeling great on the inside while glowing on the outside.

If one person has a particular query, chances are that ten others are wondering the same thing, but haven't spoken up about it yet. I want you to see if you find yourself in any of these questions and answers. Acknowledge the similarities of us human beings, and try to apply some of the answers to your own questions as they come up.

Q: When I begin losing weight I feel like I can conquer anything. I have a few burning desires on my bucket list, but cannot attempt them until I lose the last fifteen pounds. Can you help me?

A: Yes, but first we must look at why you are holding back the goals like a crutch, keeping you stuck until you lose a number of pounds. Look deeper. Let's focus on taking steps to committing to the life goals. I think that when we are so busy doing the work that will lead us to realizing our dreams, the weight will shed. There is an ease that occurs when we reverse the thinking. Anxiety about losing weight will subside because we are on to the other real life goals. Do not allow a number on a scale to dictate whether you can dance, run, learn another language, play an instrument, travel, etc.

Q: Are smoothies or juices better for us in the long run?

A: It depends on what kind of smoothie or juice you are referring to, and what you want to receive as the health benefits when ingesting them.

Green vegetable juicing is super nutrient dense without much fiber. For example, I juice kale, cabbage, leeks, spinach, parsley, cilantro, mustard greens, celery, ginger, garlic, lemon, green apple, and cucumber. In order to get 32 ounces of juice, I fill three family serving size bowls full of produce. There is no way that I could eat three family size serving bowls of fruits and vegetables! I'm talking huge! So when we condense the vitamins, minerals, and live enzymes from the large quantity of produce, the result is a very low sugar superfood in liquid form. This is also a rest for the digestive organs because there are no fibers chewed and swallowed. Thumbs up from me!

On the other hand, juicing just fruits or half fruits and vegetables creates a sugar rush to the body. The fruit sugars are absorbed slowly when it is in the whole fruit form. The skin, fibers, and flesh take time to chew and digest. This slows down the sugar absorption rate. When we chug down 32 ounces of fresh squeezed fruit juice, we may as well have had a soda and a candy bar. The body does not know the difference. Lots of fruit juice equals lots of sugar. Our bodies have only five grams of sugar floating around in the entire blood stream at any one time. Any extra that is not burned up through exertion immediately, usually turns into body fat.

Smoothies are made in the blender rather than in a juicer. The whole vegetable and fruit is pulverized with the skin and fiber included. If one is to use fruit in their beverages, this is the favorable way to do it. Again, I suggest using more vegetables than fruits, with the skin and flesh included. This also allows food matter to move through the intestines very efficiently. I call it a scrub brush for the insides. I use the bathroom frequently after a vegetable smoothie.

Once or twice a year I do a green juice fast for seven days. I think more clearly and sleep more soundly for about a month afterwards. The key is to not feel hungry. When hungry, drink the juice. When thirsty, drink the juice. I also drink my gallon of water a day, and have coffee and tea as usual. I don't count calories during the juice fast. It isn't a fast like a starvation fast. It is a fast as in not eating anything else like meats, nuts, fish, dairy, etc.

A word about juices labeled *not from concentrate*: juices on the grocery store shelves and refrigerated juices that have this label aren't always fresh squeezed and used immediately. They may be held up to a year in a giant refrigerated silo. What happens to fresh juice that sits? Usually the pulp and sediment settle to the bottom. The top becomes more watery in taste and look. Before bottling, in order to make it taste like fresh juice again, they add fruit flavoring and fruit sugars from the very fruit that it came from. So the larger companies that have fruit juices sold in cartons and bottles that are not from concentrate are sweeter and contain higher concentrates of fruit sugars. That's why I prefer to make my own. I juice my own produce, and throw a handful of fruit in for every bushel of vegetables used.

Speaking of added sugars, even nonfat milk has sugar added to it. The nonfat milk tastes relatively bland and not very milky. The dairy industry adds milk sugars to make it taste like milk again. I'll stick to my raw milk and cream, thank you.

Q: How can I ever go out to eat again? I know too much now!

A: Once you study and navigate your way around a new eating habit, whether it's the HCG protocol, ancestral eating, or just progressing towards a real foods diet, inevitably you will encounter social events. Some are at restaurants. The point of these dietary changes is to assist in your whole life, but not to take over and become your whole life. It may feel like that for a while, but trust me, after some time you will fall into a natural rhythm with what you choose to put into your mouth.

When you go into a restaurant setting, remember that you, as a guest, have the right to ask questions about exactly how your meal is being prepared. The customer also has the right to ask for modifications of food preparation. I have been a server for years and I modify meals for guests every single shift. It really is not a bother to the staff if they want to make you happy. Then you will become a loyal customer by bringing repeat business and other people with you. It really is a win-win situation.

What kinds of restaurants do I frequent? I go to seafood houses, grills, and any ethnic restaurant. I often ask the server to serve the food with all sauces on the side and lots of lemons. I request food to be made without oils unless I can be certain it is not industrial vegetable and seed oils. They may, however, slather on the butter, cream, coconut, extra virgin olive oil, etc. Restaurants and the hospitality industry are about building relationships. If the food is prepared in a manner that I can thoroughly enjoy without second guessing the nutrients and ramifications on the scale the next day, they have got me as a customer for life!

Q: Aren't oatmeal and whole grain cereals good for me?

A: While a serving of hearty O's does have just one gram of sugar per serving, the entire bowl of cereal or oatmeal is highly processed and coming from grains. Therefore that one gram of sugar turns into a bowl full of sugar during digestion because all of the carbohydrates are transformed into glucose in the blood stream. I personally do not believe it is good for the human body. I'm reminding you again that our whole body can only hold a teaspoon of sugar in the bloodstream at any one time. The insulin naturally spikes from a bowl of "healthy" whole grain cereal.

Q: I've been doing so well on my eating program for a few weeks. Now, I'm bugging my brother (who really needs to lose weight) to do this lifestyle shift with me. He refuses to listen! What do I do? I'm so frustrated. I love him, and I worry about him. He is pre-diabetic and on blood pressure medication. Help!

A: Some people cannot discuss diet openly. It's like politics and religion to some folks. They believe what they believe and you can't change their minds. Just be ready to cradle them with love and support when they are ready and open to change. The best conversation may be by your action in silence. Set the example. When they are desperate enough or scared enough, they may reach out to you. Set the table and they will come, one day...in the future.

At the same time that we are feeling the fantastic changes occurring inside of our bodies, we can't help but become zealots in expressing our commitment to our health. We may go overboard in our enthusiasm by sharing with anybody and everybody nearby. I have certainly been accused of doing so. Be careful about overdoing it and sounding preachy. Some people just don't want to hear it, even if they may benefit from eating lots of plants, seafood, and pastured animals. As my dearly departed friend Marcie used to say, "Too much cheesecake too soon..."

Q: I love my wine, beer, or cocktail at the end of a stressful day. Where does alcohol fit in to the healthy changes I have made?

A: While on the HCG protocol, alcohol is prohibited in Phase 2, and allowed on occasion in Phase 3 and beyond. On the "real life" protocol, after weight loss and change in your daily regime is established, it is, as always, personal choice.

Alcohol in the body creates the liver to focus all of its attention to processing it. Therefore it ignores the nutrients we ate alongside of the alcohol. That creates a higher amount of food that can turn into fat instead of fuel. Then we get hungry again because we did not truly nourish the body at the cellular level. So we eat again! How many times have we had a night out on the town and ended up at a diner at 2am, ravenous for our second dinner or our first breakfast?

I love a few glasses of wine or a martini on my days off. If I see that I am indulging too frequently, I give myself a week or two break from alcohol. I suggest a self check from time to time. Alcohol consumption may also aid us in giving in to spontaneous food temptations that we may have not even considered on our radar before imbibing in the stuff.

Q: I miss regular salad dressing so much. Can I ever use it again? What about "light" versions?

A: Commercial ranch and blue cheese dressings, YUMMY! I enjoy regular salad dressings too, but unfortunately they are full of additives, preservatives, chemicals, thickeners, emulsifiers, stabilizers, etc. They are not good for us. Whenever companies take ingredients out of something to make it "light," we must look at what they are replacing the full fat and full sugar versions with. Read the labels! Usually the replacement ingredients are even *worse* chemicals, additives, and artificial sweeteners. These are highly processed products which are specifically manufactured to trigger cravings. We may then begin unraveling the tightly wound yarn ball of discipline and healing from those addictions. We have worked so long and so hard to attain the health we deserve.

To me, it's just not worth it. I do not use salad dressing very often. If I do, I make it myself. Think of using Greek yogurt mixed with mineral salt, herbs, grated parmesan cheese, a little garlic, etc. There goes your ranch! I also use mustards of every variety to make dressings. I add extra virgin olive oil, lemon, varieties of vinegars, hemp oils, etc. This is the time to go a little wild and experiment with new flavor profiles because your tongue and body are fully awake and not numb with the old status quo. Just a couple of years ago I wouldn't touch a salad without fancy bottled dressing. My palate has changed and yours will too. Roll up your sleeves, open wide the cupboard doors, and reach for herbs and spices that have just been taking up space but rarely used.

Q: What is the truth about calorie counting in its relation to fat and weight loss? There are so many conflicting reports in the media?

A: Calories are a man made measure to show the energy food has for us to survive. When we are active, we can use calorie counting to show how much of that energy we use up. After the HCG protocol, I rarely use calories as a measure of my healthfulness or not. It is far more important to look at the quality of the calories than the quantity of the calories our food has. I use the macronutrient graph chart more nowadays to see if I'm getting in enough healthy fats and proteins.

Q: Do I really need supplements if I am eating this clean and healthy?

A: I compare supplements to plumbing. Do we really need indoor plumbing? You can go to the bathroom outside but why would you want to? It sure doesn't hurt to use the indoor bathroom that came with our house or apartment.

Our modern stressed out life has us multitasking at a level our ancestors didn't participate in. This affects our stress hormone cortisol, amongst others.

Stress equals cortisol. Cortisol equals fight or flight response. Fight or flight response equals holding on to fat, discomfort, and disease. The body doesn't have a homeostatic response in a stressed out environment. In this case, we cannot absorb as many particles of good nutrition from the good food we eat. Therefore good quality, pure supplements are like an insurance policy.

Many inexpensive supplements use corn starch, corn syrup, talcum powder, and cement as binders. Again, read the labels, and research what ingredients are in the supplements. I buy most of my supplements from Pure Formulas company on the internet. Many cheaper supplements are made from synthetic ingredients as well. Seek out whole food sources of concentrated supplements for the most bioavailability.

Q: What are some simple ways to de-stress? I don't have time to take yoga and meditation classes. My sleep could improve too. I toss and turn, and I am up a few times a night to use the restroom since I have increased my water intake to a gallon a day.

A: De-stressing changes the relationship to every other part of your life. Sit down to eat, even if it is in your car. Pull over to the curb, and quietly be present with your lovingly prepared delicious meal.

I sometimes park my car close to my daughter's elementary school thirty minutes or more early for her end of day pick up. I then relax, de-stress, and have my meal leisurely before the next phase of the to-do list ensues.

The peeing all day and night will lessen over time. If after six months of a gallon of water a day still has you up three times or more at night, I suggest finish the water for the day by 4pm. Then force yourself to use the restroom every hour until you go to sleep. This has helped my coaching clients tremendously. My personal experience is that after three weeks of the water intake, I went back to my normal routine of urination.

Melatonin under the tongue will help prepare the body to rest in a peaceful way. It is a natural hormone our brain releases to let us know it is time to go to sleep. We release less melatonin in modern times due to artificial light when the sun goes down.

When I toss and turn, I immediately get up and put cherry melatonin, one milligram sublingually. Within twenty minutes I am peacefully sleepy and ready to rest. The next morning I feel like I had a delicious sleep. That's the only way I can describe it.

Another simple way to de-stress is a one minute (yes, sixty seconds only!) meditation. I sit anywhere, alone and close my eyes. I slowly count up to ten and back down to one in my head six times. Then I open my eyes. That extreme focus and intent on only the one digit at a time is also an extreme focus and intention of letting everything else go for a minute, literally. Do this a couple of times a day. In a few weeks you may go all crazy and attempt two minutes!

Q: I gained five pounds over the holidays. Do I have to dramatically reduce my calories or go on HCG all over again?

A: Absolutely not! If you have stabilized in your new weight set point for about six months after any weight loss protocol, chances are that your body is comfortable with the new, lower set point. Here is what has worked for me: I cut out all dairy, alcohol, fruit, and nuts for a couple of weeks. I eat very clean, lots of raw and cooked vegetables, seafood, and fish. That's it. Keep in mind that I do not eat grains anyway. If you normally eat grains, I would cut them out as well for the two weeks. See if this helps, and please send me feedback on your experience.

Q: Can I live on HCG forever? I eat so clean and have no cravings or set backs when I am on the hormone. I do not cheat, and frankly, I am afraid to go off of HCG. Help!

A: Wake up! This protocol was designed to get obese people to a clean eating state. It was designed to be used until there was no more abnormal fat on the body. It was designed to be long enough in time to build new habits that can be sustained without torturing us once the HCG protocol is over. After a new metabolism is established, there should be no fear moving into Phase 3 or 4. The conscious effort required to maintain the new you is all YOU. The hormone won't work if you take it your whole life and eat a low calorie diet forevermore. Why? Your body will eventually run out of extra fat, and then the body will turn to muscle for fuel. Your muscles will break down, and you will feel fatigue all the time. You will feel lethargic, and have memory loss. Your joints will ache without the lubrication that fat provides.

The brain is over two thirds fat. Fats and cholesterol have a function in the brain and body or we would not have it at all inside of us! The human body is a remarkable functional machine. The body has all the answers. Everything in the human body has its purpose. After we have lost the excess fat on the HCG program we must add good healthy fats back into the diet. Fats carry the nutrients from other foods into the blood stream more easily. Good fats keep us fuller longer. The wrong kinds of fats and oils (hydrogenated, trans-fats, margarines, vegetable oils) combined with sugar and processed ingredients will make us gain weight and fat. The healthy fats will not. Preservatives and additives that are meant to add and preserve on the grocery store shelves will add and preserve on the hips, thighs, and abdomen. I was proof of that.

The HCG protocol is not meant to be a yoyo diet either. We cannot go on and off of it every couple of months. The gorging days on HCG may not be used as an excuse to follow it again. "Ooh, I get to eat whatever I want for two days. Then I will be *good* because I know the weight will come right off." It is not about that sort of mind set. The HCG protocol was designed to get us into a new mind set for life.

So, do not fool yourself. Do the work with your passion toward your goals and carry on with the new lifestyle. You are stronger than you give yourself credit for. Just ask those around you.

Q: I see homeopathic HCG all over the internet. Will that work just as well as the prescription kind?

A: No! Homeopathic HCG has no HCG in it. It is mostly water and vitamins. The FDA is trying to shut down all homeopathic operations. It is illegal to sell HCG over the counter. We must get a prescription from a physician or order from overseas reputable pharmacies. If one loses weight on the homeopathic HCG, it is because they are starving themselves. Eventually the muscles will atrophy, the cravings will be unbearable, and the protocol will fail.

Q: I'm not rich and afford to buy all organic produce, wild caught seafood, and grass fed animal products. Do I have to abandon the idea of finally getting super healthy and losing weight?

A: No! I am a server in a restaurant and am not wealthy at all. If something is on sale, is organic, and it's reasonable, I will buy it. Trader Joe's grocery store has a multitude of goodies that are organic and very inexpensive. Local farmers' markets are another good option because the produce there is uber fresh and they take the middle man away, making it affordable. I think eating organic will become more affordable for the general public when we stop spending money on regular cookies, pies, cakes, pastries, breads, cereals, rice, crackers, pasta, chips, candy, tortillas, etc.

My pediatrician said that 100 years ago nothing was labeled organic, but almost everything was organic anyway. Today the organic farmers and food manufacturers have to pay a lot of money to have the right to stamp the word organic on their products. They have stiff inspections as well. That is a couple of reasons why organic food is more expensive.

Even if you do not buy organic food while on a health quest, your health and wellness will improve with the protocols described here. Eating non-starchy vegetables, fresh fish, pastured animals, and fruit on occasion is a huge improvement over the Standard American Diet. Just by eliminating sugars, artificial sugar substitutes, grains, and packaged refined foods will change our health and our future for the better.

Q: Artificial sweeteners are zero calories. Can I use any kind on my departure from added sugar?

A: Let's get one thing clear my friends. Artificial sweeteners are chemicals. They are not the same thing as plant based, zero calorie sweeteners. There are many of both kinds of sugar substitutes out there. Here is a quick overview of the more popular ones:

SACCHARIN is an artificial sweetener with a sulfa base. It has a slight metallic aftertaste. Saccharin may cause nausea, diarrhea, skin problems, or other common allergic symptoms. It has even been linked to bladder cancer. My body reacts to saccharin as if I have had soda. I use the restroom repeatedly every hour. It makes me more thirsty afterwards, and then I tend to crave salty things.

ASPARTAME is made from Phenylalanine, aspartic acid, and methanol gas. It also has a slightly bitter or metallic aftertaste. Side effects may include headaches, memory loss, anxiety, heart palpitations, and weight gain! What? Weight gain? Yes, the body thinks it is enjoying sugar, and may spike the insulin as if you had sugar anyway.

SUCRALOSE is a substance made by chlorinating sugar. The chemical structure of the type of chlorine in the table top sucralose is the type of chlorine that is banned in the pesticide named DDT! People who use sucralose have reported headaches, muscle aches, cramps, diarrhea, dizziness, and inflammation.

Sucralose can impact the immune system, the liver, and the kidneys.

STEVIA is a plant based zero calorie sweetener. It grows in South America and Central America. The leaves are dried and powdered. Some brands do have a metallic or bitter aftertaste. Some people report that after a while they do not notice it. Low doses of stevia have been used for years in Japan for lowering high LDL cholesterol (the bad kind) and controlling type 2 diabetes.

LUO HAN GUO is the extract from the Chinese monk fruit. It has been used for centuries in Asia as a sweet tea for sore throats, flu, and joint pain. The Japanese have crystallized it into a brown, sugar-like substance called Lakanto. It is zero calorie, and has no effect on the glycemic index. It has no bitter or metallic aftertaste. Some American companies are using the sugar substitute in their health food products now. Some newer versions of the sugar substitute have added corn starch to the ingredients list. As always, I suggest reading labels. Lakanto released a white sugar version recently, but for me, the golden brown version is more authentic to the sugar taste.

XYLITOL is a low calorie sweetener extracted from the bark of the birch tree. Some companies extract other hard wood barks and plants as well. It looks, tastes, and bakes like white sugar. It does have calories, about 9-10 per teaspoon, but will not spike the insulin levels in the body, as it is very low on the glycemic index. There is no aftertaste at all. Over consumption of xylitol can cause gas, diarrhea, and bloating in some cases.

Artificial sweeteners can stimulate the appetite and cravings, therefore making us eat more than we may need. It creates in our body the supposition that we took in more calories than we actually did (from sugar), so after a while when the digestion system gets the message from the brain that we didn't actually eat a lot of calories, we physically need to fill that void. Artificial chemical sweeteners disrupt the insulin and leptin receptors. Our metabolism gets confused. Some artificial sweeteners have chemicals in them that stimulate and excite the brain cells so much, that they are called excitotoxins. First they excite the brain cells, then they kill them off.

Personally, I use Lakanto golden brown variety and Xyla white for my sugar alternatives. Now I am experimenting with coffee and tea without any sweetener, just cinnamon sprinkled in or lemon. I have had no side effects from either sweetener.

Q: What is it with MSG? I see it everywhere!

A: As a server, I hear people saying they are allergic to MSG all the time without knowing exactly what it is. It is a food additive and a flavor enhancer. MSG stands for Monosodium Glutamate. What many folks do not know is that there are many sneaky names in the food industry for MSG. Anything on an ingredient list that has the word glutamate in it has MSG in it. Other words for MSG include autolyzed yeast, hydrolyzed yeast, maltodextrin, "flavoring," soy protein extract, and a host of others. Look up the complete list for MSG on the internet. You will be surprised. Many low fat items have MSG added to them to make the food taste like their full fat counterparts. MSG is another excitotoxin. I need all of my brain cells to write this book, and to share my world! How about you?

Q: I thought I was the fittest and most committed one in the gym. Then this teeny, tiny, totally ripped woman walked into the room, and my self esteem plummeted. What gives?

A: This is a classic case of doing your best versus being the best. Showing up and working mind, body, and spirit toward your health and healing goals are huge steps to undertake. You are here and doing your best. You are reading this book for a reason. Honestly looking at yourself, the journey, and the transformation occurring right now is what counts. You are doing your best. Say this ten times and be happy where you are right now. I guarantee there will always be someone leaner and fitter than you. I also guarantee there will always be someone larger and less fit than you. That larger person may have felt defeated in the same way you did when she or he walked into the room. The smaller and fitter woman or man may have been *you* six months ago. We cannot figure out everybody else's pathway to *here* and *now*, so just focus on you. Do *you*. Be *you*.

Q: There are so many fat burners out there. How do I know which ones really work?

A: After spending lots of money on fat burners purchased at the local pharmacy or health food store with no results except very expensive pee, I decided to use pharmaceutical grade fat burners with no fillers or binders. I use gelatin capsules that do not contain soy. After losing fat and weight, I reduced my collection to three that seemed to have the best effects on me. I take cinnamon, cayenne pepper, and carnitine tartrate. Two out of the three are food based so they are more bioavailable than synthetic fat burners.

Carnitine tartrate powder is an amino acid that supports fat burning and energy levels. Cinnamon regulates blood sugars throughout the day and reduces sugar cravings because there are less dips in energy. Cayenne pepper increases the heat in the body and revs up metabolism. The three fat burners together can lower cholesterol, balance sugar levels in the blood, and improve circulation. I stopped taking anything else because when I reduced my supplements, these were the deciding factors in my stabilization of weight and mood. When I experimented by taking away the synthetic fat burners, there was no difference in my health or my perception of my health. Again, read the labels. Products with less fillers and binders are better for us, and will be better absorbed by the body.

Q: What is intermittent fasting?

A: Intermittent fasting is going without food for a period of time just like our ancestors did. Some methods use a twenty four hour fast a few times a week. Other methods allow an eight hour window every day in which to eat meals. If there are enough good fats ingested during the meals, there is little to no hunger during the time one is not eating. My own intermittent fasting habit occurred unconsciously and spontaneously. Because of my work schedule, I eat dinner around 8pm to 9pm on the work evenings. I am not hungry for food until about 2pm each day. I work out in a fasted state (except coffee with a tablespoon or two of cream), and drink close to a gallon of water by noon. This seems to keep my mind sharp and my focus on my workout very precise as far as technique is concerned. My reading and podcasts I have heard that speak about intermittent fasting support my personal experience. It also is a way to burn body fat efficiently.

Even the HCG protocol has intermittent fasting built into it naturally without naming it so. Breakfast is coffee, tea, or water. We eat our first solid food at lunch. That is about a twelve to eighteen hour window without food. Our bodies turn to its stored fat as fuel during this time. Again, I give to kudos to Dr. Simeons!

Q: How have the nuclear disaster in Japan and pollution in general affected our seafood and fish supply? Isn't it too risky to eat fish?

A: All living things have exposure to and accumulation of toxins from the environment. We are a product of our modern world. The longer an animal is alive, the longer amount of time one has to accumulate the toxins. The larger the animal, the more pollution one absorbs. Research shows that there are no serious poisons we should be overly concerned with. As a result of the nuclear disaster, Japan now has a stricter guideline than the world has ever had, ever, as far as radioactivity and metal toxicity in the seafood and fish supply.

We humans are very resilient. Fish and seafood are nutrient rich and healthy, especially if they are not fed grains on a fish farm. Smaller fish are less likely to have metals and toxicity in them compared to larger species. Bottom dwellers and bi-valve seafood like clams, oysters, mussels, etc. are extremely rich in zinc and other minerals that our body needs. Shrimp shells and fish bones are calcium rich, if you can stomach them. I love collecting the kids' shrimp shells when we go out to eat, and hoard them for myself!

Q: What is GMO? What is GEO?

A: Genetically modified organisms are nicknamed GMO. It usually means crops that have been made resistant to pesticides. So when we spray the crops, the vegetables, fruits, and grains will grow while the pesty insects are killed.

Genetically engineered organisms are nicknamed GEO. It usually means foods that are engineered to be a new kind of food. An example of this is a pluot. It is a plum and an apricot cross bred to make a new fruit with flavors of both original fruits. When deciding what type of produce to buy, we must consider the earth's environment and ways to sustain our Mother Earth. Usually non-GMO crops will be grown in more nutrient dense soil, but that is not always the case. That may result in more nutrient rich produce.

One problem in the United States with GMO foods is that there are no labeling laws for GMO crops. If an item at the grocery store specifically says non-GMO, then we can reasonably think that it is true. Other than that, there are no guarantees. Some organic crops have become GMO crops because of cross pollination in the air. If organic farms are near other farms that grow GMO crops, there is a chance they will become pollinated with GMO pollen.

Knowledge is power. Here is a list of the most common GMO crops in the USA:

- soy
- corn
- wheat
- alfalfa
- papaya
- canola (rapeseed)

- cotton
- sugar beets
- zucchini
- yellow squash

Recently I received a letter in the mail from my health provider. It stated that we should stay away from GMO foods. It encouraged people to stay away from GMO foods because the long term effects have not been studied yet. Eliminating those foods from our diet can resolve aches and pains associated with inflammation. These are the most common types of complaints at the doctors' offices.

There are many more questions and answers than I could possibly include here. Please view my website, blog, YouTube channel, and Facebook page for weekly updates on queries. As you go through your journey to a happier and healthier version of yourself, do not hesitate to ask questions and seek out the answers. Do not allow the questions to keep piling up in your head to the point where you can't move forward until you have your questions answered. Questions will continuously pop up our whole lives. That is the fabulous nature of the brilliant human mind!

Chapter Ten

THEIR STORIES

I love to tell stories. I feel like stories help us to understand the meanings behind the points we are trying to get across to someone. When you read the following stories of my clients, friends, and family, see if any of their predicaments are similar to yours. If you can easily imagine yourself in their position, acknowledge it, and figure out how you would react. Would it be similar or different after recognizing that your feet could easily be in their shoes?

Most of my clients become my friends. I'm not only their mentor and coach, but also their confidante. We are intertwined in so many areas of each others' lives. They are sharing their mental, physical, and spiritual struggles with me. I share my personal weaknesses with them too, in order to make them see that their crutches are not theirs alone. We are stronger together.

Emma~

Emma had a desire to stop eating junk foods and carbohydrates. She didn't know anything about grains and sugars making her overweight and bloated. She just knew what she liked and had a cultural connection to many unhealthy foods. Family traditions are important to all of us. Unfortunately, for many of us, that revolves around foods that are high in processed oils, starches, and sugars. Emma had a love affair with diet cola too.

One day, she posted on a social network that she was a piggy because she ate pizza and garlic bread at the same meal. She insulted herself on the internet in front of the whole world! She deserved self love, not self loathing. I saw that post as a cry for help. I offered my guidance, and it was accepted. She promised to abide by new criteria for eating. For thirty days Emma did not consume bad dietary fats, sugar, artificial sweeteners, or grains. She increased her water to a gallon a day. She reported to me a month later that she had lost weight and her energy was renewed. Her soda consumption remained slim to none. Her family and friends noticed something shiny, sparkly, and different about her. I called it her superior self coming out of the shadows. Recently she has embarked upon green vegetable juicing as a way to increase micronutrients in her diet. Bravo!

Arthur~

Arthur is a devout Christian. He told me that one day God and Jesus helped him give up alcohol, drugs, and homelessness, cold turkey. I saw him struggle with sweets whenever our paths would intersect. One day I mustered up the courage to ask him why he could give up drugs and alcohol with the Lord's assistance, but cave in to sugar and refined carbohydrates. I asked him to pray just as deeply for help in this area.

Soon after, he and his wife watched the documentary film featuring Joe Cross. It is called *FAT, SICK, AND NEARLY DEAD.* It chronicles a journey of an ill, overweight, Australian executive through his 60 day green juice fast. Joe's illnesses cleared up, and he lost 100 pounds during the process. The film had an emotional impact on Arthur. He told me afterwards that he and his wife were planning on juicing with vegetables as a meal replacement for one meal a day. After that commitment felt comfortable, Arthur moved to two meals a day. He also increased his water tremendously. Whenever he sees me, he rushes to get a glass of water. I remind him that water intake is of the utmost importance when changing to a healthier lifestyle.

Arthur is certainly on his way. He falls off the food wagon from time to time, but we are all human. He stands up, dusts himself off, and walks tall and proud towards his healthier future.

Food addiction is not like alcohol and drug addiction. When we give up drugs and alcohol, the goal is to give it up completely. If we give up food completely, we perish and die. I believe this makes it even more difficult to evolve into superior habits with food. That is why I give kudos, huge congratulations, honor, and respect to those who finally do develop consistent eating habits that feed their brains, bodies, and spirits.

Jessica~

Jessica had been withholding patience, respect, attention, and support from her own body for a long time. She loved herself, but did not know how to physically show that love to herself. She tried different cleanses and juicing techniques over the years, but seemed to bounce back into processed foods and sugary alcoholic beverages soon after.

Stress reared its head from a very young age. She dealt with the family and home stress through episodes of bulimia. The same thirty pounds came and went numerous times. In her head, she knew what to do to correct the problem. Making the brain-heart-body connection daily was an overwhelming challenge. Jessica asked me to coach her in a 43 day round of HCG.

During the protocol, Jessica learned what foods her body needed more of and what foods her body no longer craved. She gave up alcohol completely. Her resistance to exercise fell by the wayside. Jessica has actively been hiking, taking Pilates classes, and experimenting in new and unusual fitness classes. There is a renewed self confidence and self trust. She has said YES to herself and YES to life.

Danny~

Danny is a gifted massage therapist. He is intuitive in his healing and closes his eyes when he massages clients. When I first started going to him for my own massage needs, I was in the first thirty days of my HCG protocol. He watched me melt right before his eyes in the months that followed.

Over the years we have talked deeply about nutrition, fitness, and life goals. Eventually Danny asked me to guide him on his own Wellness From Within journey. Witnessing my transformation first hand motivated him to do something about his obesity.

The first week I took him shopping at an inexpensive produce market and a high end organic market. We swapped out his oils and nuts. We bought raw cheeses and healthy grain free snacks. Then I walked him through the Guide to Wellness from Within..

I feel like a proud mama! It takes a lot of courage to own up to yourself *and* to someone else that you know what you have been doing thus far has not been in your best health interest. Danny has been consistent in drinking a gallon of water a day. Danny fell off the wagon a couple of times in the ten weeks. After just two bites of pizza, he called me on the phone and shared that those two bites actually made him sick to his stomach. For the first time in his life he was tuning in to what his body asked for. It did not ask for pizza.

I am so happy that he entrusted me with his body goals and his future health. Danny tells me that he feels so much better physically these days. His struggle is with the rest of his family. They say they want to eat real, whole foods along with him, but they consistently buy packaged and processed foods. They overfill the pantry, cupboards, counters, and top of the refrigerator with temptations that Danny must resist. Every day is a battle, but he is winning the war.

Wendy~

Wendy works for a self help and transformative company. They host intensive, weeklong therapy sessions where true personal change can happen. At first I thought she may have tried to reach the wrong person. How could I help her? She has coaching available at her fingertips.

She asked me to coach her on a 26 day round of HCG because she heard my story and advice when I was a guest on the HCG Body for Life podcast. Wendy said she had been trying to reach me for a long time. She felt my messages of continued health and maintenance had concrete advice and spiritual wisdoms that resonated with her. She had done HCG before and had cheated every few days. She had gained and lost the same 10 to 15 pounds a few times. Her desire was to stop the yoyo dieting and finally be in a place where she could not obsess about her size. She wanted to breathe and be free!

Our work together has been very honest and fulfilling for both of us. She realized that her cheating while on the HCG was a reflection of her bucking authority. What a real breakthrough. Wendy is inspiring to me because she never gives up. The striving to better her life, to let go of the past, and to follow new rules that she makes herself is uncharted territory. Go Wendy, go!

Ricky~

Ricky was one of my biggest skeptics. He came to one of my wellness workshops in the middle of the nine week series. He was 30 pounds overweight. He had severe allergies and asthma his entire adult life. The allergies and asthma kept him from moving around very often or very well. Regular exercise was not available to him in his current condition. Ricky had constant constipation for ten years, caused by his medications.

He was jaded to say the least, but he stayed with me for the entire workshop, asked questions and proceeded to promise to do the first step, the gallon of water a day for a month (he chose the slower promises to himself rather than the weekly shifts, which is completely fine with me).

Ricky is in his 60s and is a talented painter and comedian. He made jokes about the Guide to Wellness from Within that got the whole room rolling with laughter, but I was well aware that his humor was an attempt to cover up his fear.

Fast forward thirty days: Ricky has lost 10 pounds without changing anything else in his diet. He is more energized to complete his honey-do list that the family gives him. He is clearer with his thoughts, and his relationships with his sons have improved. His battle with constipation is over. Ricky walks an hour every day around his neighborhood. He now is my biggest supporter, and is ready to take on step two, removing wheat and gluten from his diet. He is excited to see where the steps take him, now that he has seen proof that it works!

Vivian~

Vivian and I met in a silent, sweaty hot yoga class. She chatted with me after class, when usually people crawl to the door like limp rags. At age 83, Vivian had been doing hot yoga for years, took an eight year break, and then came back. She still worked, drove, and took care of a house with an extensive garden. Vivian and I talked every few days. One morning she shared that she had type 2 diabetes. She was shaped like an apple but not fat by any means. I was surprised that she had diabetes. Vivian asked me to meet her at the library and walk her through the Guide to Wellness from Within. We met and discussed the steps to help shift her eating and drinking, but she was already doing most of the program on her own volition. There were only a few corrections to be tackled. She took notes and took me seriously.

I checked in with her every few weeks and we have had some great conversations full of light and laughter. There is a great mutual respect there. I respect Vivian because of her agility and her ability to be fully active and vibrant as a senior in today's world. Many folks her age are slowing way down. She respects me because I was willing to help her and take time away from my children and jobs in order to give her the tools that she could use practically to change her health for the better.

I'm beaming with pride at her progress. Vivian has reported to me that after just three months of using the guide, her doctor told her that her diabetes is completely gone. She continues to test her blood sugar levels with a glucose monitor and is sweetly satisfied that her numbers are now in the optimum range every day. Vivian is an inspiration to the rest of the world because she shows us that you *can* teach an old dog new tricks after all. It is never too late, especially when the results are proof that when one does the work, the work leads to measurable success.

Chapter Eleven

YOUR STORY

*D*ear Readers,

I have given you an arsenal to go into battle against the mainstream American diet, the media deception, and general misinformation. I have given you tools to face your past choices with dignity and clarity. You can change your life now. The next chapter belongs to you. You have a natural birthright given to you from the universe when you came into the world. To be healthy, happy, vital, clear, vigorous, robust, and to meet challenges head on is your birthright. Take it and go forward on that path that is your personal journey toward vigorous health and wellness. See this learning process as a gateway to your next big thing: YOU.

I have shared with you my story of transformation and the burning desire I have to help spread the truth about our food choices. I hereby pass the baton to you.

The body and the mind changing for the better is not magic. Change is the response to your efforts applied repeatedly. Never say, "I give up, I'm going backwards towards potato chips, donuts, and fried chicken." Never say, "I give up," then stopping by the corner store for taquitos, nachos, hot dogs, and a slushie. By this point in your journey you should feel sick to your stomach just visualizing all of that!

I used to be a jack of all trades and master of none. I didn't really have one particular passion or path that I loved. I loved doing so many things. If you are like me, in that sort of boat, I say be a master of what you *don't* want in your life. Start there.

Human beings are always reaching for something. Sometimes that reaching is a distraction from sitting with what we are feeling at that very moment. We give up alcohol and drugs, and faithfully attend the twelve step programs. While we are there we incessantly reach for the coffee, donuts, and cigarettes. We reach for new things to replace the old things instead of allowing the space to be just that...space. We attend a yoga class, and when we are to rest completely still on our backs in dead man's pose, we reach to wipe our sweat or tear drop tickling our skin, running down towards our ear. Why can't we be present and still? We reach for the towel, the water bottle, etc. Whatever we reach for, we can change that and internalize it. Reach for yourself. Sit with the depth of discomfort for a few seconds longer rather than ignoring what just came up within your soul spot. These are the seeds of true change. It happens one millisecond at a time.

Relationships to our food are reflections of our connections to other human beings. As our relationship to the food changes, our relationships to every other part of our lives change. We can be free to be who we really are with our friends and family. We can begin creating more clear and honest connections and traditions. When that happens, we will feel more connected to the whole world and know we are part of something greater. Our future will seem open and vibrant.

In my family, we have a tradition of thank you bites. If facing a new and unusual food that is nutrient rich, but unfamiliar, we all take thank you bites to try it out. We feel connected to the labor and energy it took to bring the food from the fields to our mouths. We thank the sun for shining down upon the farm, the rain for watering the produce and animals, the farmers for their hard labor, the delivery system that brought the food to the grocery store, the chef who cooked the food, and the person serving the food seamlessly to our table. These thank you bites bring gratitude from our hearts, and more often than not we discover a new flavor profile that we enjoy. I like to call it truth in sustenance. It brings food to a sacred level. What is your sacred food? What is your food tradition and story that elevates your soul and your connection to others?

Important to the plan of action for any long term life change are **fuel, focus,** and **endurance.** They work together to get results.

Your **fuel** is this book and the foods you choose to eat going forward. It is also the fire within you that says, "I got this!" See yourself in the future-present instead of in a state of want. Want creates more wanting and a belief that you are in lack. Fuel yourself with gratefulness for the healthy, optimal body and mind. We humans can talk ourselves into almost anything and everything. How many times have we seen an "okay" looking outfit on sale for 80% off and bought it, talking ourselves into the purchase because it looked "great," and the price couldn't be beat? Then it sat in the back of our closet for a year until we gave it to charity. Yes, talk to yourself. Talk yourself into the body and life of your dreams. Say, "Thank you for my healthy, fit, lean, and strong body!" This is the fuel.

Focus is where you dig your heels in and allow those things and people attempting to distract you from your goals to fall away to the side like a set of dominoes. Does the family support or sabotage you? How can the family say they support me when they constantly offer me food that is clearly not on my program? "Just one bite!" I heard again and again. "It won't kill you!" The sabotage may not be intentional, but it is sabotage nonetheless. Being extremely clear about where you want to go with your health is a way to keep your focus intact. Write it down on a small piece of paper and place the paper somewhere where you can see it every day.

Your focus can be fine tuned by helping someone else. Getting out of your own head sometimes is a good thing. If you volunteer to coach someone else, you become a role model for them. They will be looking to you for guidance. You will be less likely to make deprecating choices. It becomes a karmic circle of loving yourself into success as you are loving the other person that you are mentoring. There is a higher level of accountability when someone is counting on you. Your sense of focus is heightened.

Endurance is the power to stick it out. We build endurance by making it through these twenty four hours with our fuel and focus in place. Then we do it again tomorrow...and so on. Old way of thinking: "Oh, I have such a long way to go. How am I ever going to last? There is so much to remember and so much to give up!" New way of thinking: "I can eliminate one food that does not serve my higher purpose. Tomorrow, I can eliminate another food that does not serve my higher purpose." We can build upon that. Instead of again thinking in terms of lack and that which you cannot have, think of switching it out. For example, switch out soy, canola, corn, peanut, and cottonseed oil for coconut oil. You have just simplified your grocery list, saved money, time, and served your higher purpose.

We are on earth for a limited time. Even our long term goals are really short term goals in the grand scheme of things. It is how we carry ourselves and what we choose to partake in every moment that will make a difference in our health and happiness. It will also make a difference in the legacy we leave behind. If we want to be truly healthy and balanced in mind, body, and spirit, we must change our behavior and then the rest will follow naturally, eventually. Self trust is key too. Trust the fact that you have arrived here and now, reading this book at exactly the right time in your life. I have seen the perfect body out there...and it is mine. I have seen the perfect body out there...and it is yours. At any stage in our journey our bodies have provided us with our heart, legs, arms, breath, and life. Be grateful for your perfect body. I am.

I have implemented these tools of fuel, focus, and endurance into my own life. That is what brought me to this moment right now, to be able to return the love multiple times and pay it forward.

I'm not special. I mean, I am extraordinarily special, but not any more special than you. I'm a normal human being going through the regular routines of any active mother, wife, and employee. I'm extremely busy catering to everybody's needs while taking care of me, too. I am a server (waitress in old-school talk) at a busy restaurant that has food all around, all of the time. I am constantly offered leftovers, tastings, alcohol, food training, and food gifts brought in by coworkers. I have plenty of opportunities to indulge in the wrong foods and the right foods every single day.

I must love myself more than the momentary dip into foods that don't serve my higher purpose. You have the same health and food choices as I do. As I said, I am not that special.

I compare my body to a vehicle. I would not purchase a Rolls Royce and fill up the gas tank with the cheapest fuel. When I get a premium machine like that, I would only consider the highest quality fuel. The human body is the most precious machine we will ever be given the opportunity to take care of. I strongly suggest that we give it premium fuel so that it may perform beyond our wildest expectations. Just like researching and planning before buying that luxury car, our superior food journey can be premeditated and deliberate. To be a star in our own show that is this life, we must provide our bodies with stellar products.

If the media based diet industry of pills, powders, replacement shakes, and prepackaged processed meals truly worked, long term, once and for all, we would witness the end of the obesity epidemic. We would all be fit looking and feeling wonderful most of the time. Our health markers and blood tests would prove them to be successful. That has not happened yet. That is a fantasy. Put the diet pill down and give your power back to yourself.

We are not meant to be at war with ourselves, especially not over food. When we give in to spontaneous temptation unconsciously, we are giving our power away. While on any protocol that enhances our health and power, if we suddenly say, "Screw it!" and stuff the highly processed chocolate chip muffin in our mouths, we have just given our power to that muffin. Then the muffin sits in our stomachs, we feel guilty, and maybe not so energized. Then the muffin makes its way through our digestive system and we use the restroom. Literally and figuratively, we have turned our power to crap and flushed it down the toilet. Take your power back.

The answers won't be found in yet another new "clinically proven" magic diet pill or potion. The answers lie in your own head, heart, and hands. Take action for yourself. Research, read, and ask questions of the experts in this field. If we realistically and honestly take care of ourselves, we have the opportunity to take even greater care of our children. If we are not jumping in to our best life possible, we may not even be around or capable of caring for our next generation. I know I sound like a commercial and it seems a little cliché. I feel your heads nodding in agreement, while at the same time, slightly resistant to drastic change. I was in your shoes a few short years ago. I was trying to juggle two jobs, two kids, an insane workout schedule, friends, family, and a husband. I did not have time for me. I did not have time or money to cook clean and green, read labels, and prepare Paleo convenience foods.

So it is basically about prioritizing. Do you love yourself? Do you love yourself enough to streamline the excess stuff in your life so that you may be exuberant and full of the extra energy that the streamlining produces?

The money for clean and green foods comes when we stop purchasing grains, sugars, and packaged processed foods. The money will come when we stop buying very expensive baby gifts when we know the baby prefers the pretty wrapping paper and bow the gift arrived in. The money will come when we don't have to take the kids to the doctor for yet another cold, flu, or allergic reaction, probably caused by undiagnosed food sensitivities.

Then, with that extra time away from the doctor's office, we can go to the park and play with our children because we have time, money, and energy! Being energized and having fun play dates with my kids makes me happy. Having hiking and running dates with friends on my days off have replaced cocktails and all-you-can-eat pasta at the Italian eateries (before noon, at that!). Move more, lift heavy things, play, and laugh more. The answers are there, in your happy spot.

Your journey, like mine, may have begun with being in a mid-life funk, being slightly disgusted every time you look in the mirror, being tired despite the good food and exercise you do, despite the vitamins and energy drinks you consume. Now it may be to the point in your journey where you switch it up to how you feel is more important than how you look. Looking good is a result of the feeling good. It is a side effect. It is the icing on the cake (so to speak). As a society, we continue to place too much emphasis on how our bodies look rather than on how our bodies perform. We can look fabulous and still die of something tomorrow. Simply commit to healthy choices. This much is in our control. I pray you have enhanced health. I pray you have enhanced performance in your daily life activities and goals. I pray you have enhanced longevity as a result of the action you take based upon the ideas presented here.

So here we are at the end of this book. My prescription for you is to mix equal parts spirituality, hard work, dedication, and dreams fulfilled. Sprinkle a lot of potential powder on top. Put it all in the blender, give it a whirl, and drink a cup each morning. This is your recipe for change. Realize your superior self.

MEAL IDEAS

*T*he creations I throw together every day are delicious and nourish the whole person. For the most part, I do not measure because I love to experiment and be resourceful with what I have in the house. I refrain from using sugar and grains, and I embrace good dietary fats. All of the meals here are appropriate for the HCG diet and beyond. Use these meal ideas as a launching pad for your superior self. Any meal here is based on high quality, real, whole foods. They are nutritious for any healthy eating strategy. I encourage you to experiment and have fun!

HCG Phase 2 Friendly Meals (and beyond)

- Sear lobster tails in coconut oil, basil, garlic, and pink Himalayan salt. Sauté spinach and burn some cabbage. Splash some balsamic vinegar on top of veggies.

- Steam Swai fish in an inch of lemon water or chicken broth. Add a side of raw chipotle sauerkraut and steamed kale. Top with sugar free salsa and spicy mustard.

- Sear tilapia fish in coconut oil and gluten free tamari sauce. Add lots of garlic purée on top. For a side dish, sauté red cabbage with caramelized onions over raw spinach. Add lots of spicy mustard and Paleo BBQ sauce.

- Sear Brussels sprouts in a tiny bit of coconut oil. If you burn them, they taste like artichoke hearts! Add Phase 2 protein.

- Chop raw celery, flake red snapper fish, toss into Herdez sugar free salsa. Splash raw apple cider vinegar on the top.

- Steam cod in chicken broth with chives, asparagus, and broccoli stems. Add lemongrass and paprika to taste.

- Line a platter with white fish carpaccio (yes that's raw), grapefruit wedges, capers, and lemon wedges.

- Stir fry Miracle noodles (fettuccine or angel hair style) in coconut oil. Stir in garlic, lemon, onions, scallions, shrimp, steamed tomatoes and spinach. Add a little bit of coconut oil, salt and pepper. (Miracle noodles are a calorie free glucomannan noodle originating from Japan.)

- Sear mushrooms, green zucchini, purple cabbage, and celery with a tiny bit of coconut oil and balsamic vinegar. Add garlic, lemon, Lakanto, salt and pepper.

- Add crab and spinach to an egg white omelet.

- Toss arugula and raw mushrooms with cucumbers. Add balsamic vinegar, lemon, salt, pepper, curry powder. Pan sear a chicken breast with a teaspoon of coconut oil and caramelize garlic cloves.

- Blend in a high speed blender: cooked kale, cauliflower, cabbage, onion, ginger, garlic and broccoli. Add a little salt, pepper, and curry paste. The green one from Mae Ploy is Phase 2 appropriate. It makes a green vegetable, creamy soup.

- Pan fry cilantro, cabbage, and fennel in a lemony Lakanto broth. Add chives and any white fish. Cilantro is a good blood purifier and pulls heavy metal toxins out of your body.

- Sear boneless chicken breast with baby bok choy and purple cabbage. Add Himalayan salt and curry powder. Drizzle coconut oil on top.

- Sauté 99 percent fat free ground chicken, tomatoes, mushrooms, broccoli, zucchini, onions, garlic, basil, oregano, and thyme. Add to giant green cabbage cups.

HCG Phase 3 Friendly Meals (and beyond)

- Grill onions, chili peppers, nopales cactus, and shrimp. Add avocado slices.

- Toss raw spinach, pickled cranberries, raw goat cheese, extra virgin first cold pressed olive oil, radishes, hearts of palm, hearts of artichoke, and pastured shredded chicken breast. Season to taste.

- Mix canned clams in water, sardines in brine, mushrooms, broccoli slaw, and tomatoes. Top with mayonnaise made with olive oil, not soy oil or canola oil.

- Make your own shrimp cocktail with Herdez brand salsa, chopped onions, scallions, parsley, cilantro, garlic, and limes. Serve with radishes on the side. Add avocado.

- Sear Brussels sprouts until blackened a little. Toss in hot red pepper slivers, caramelized onions, and raw milk Parmesan cheese. Top with seared scallops in MCT oil.

- Make ground turkey meatballs stuffed with home minced basil and garlic. For the sauce, sauté garlic and Lakanto sprinkled into diced tomatoes. Add green onion and raw milk cheddar cheese. Wrap up in large lettuce leaves or coconut wraps.

- Pizza: Steam and hand crush cauliflower. Put in between towels and squeeze out moisture. Mix with raw eggs, raw hard cheeses, and garlic. Press in cookie sheet lined with foil and olive oil. Bake 25 minutes at 400 degrees. Pull out and add raw cheeses, pesto, sugar free red sauce, and any other proteins and/or vegetables. Place back in the oven for 30 minutes more until edges are crispy and the top and bottom are golden brown.

- Sear salmon in grapeseed oil. Top with pesto sauce. On the side, stew tomatoes in apple cider vinegar and Lakanto. Add raw sauerkraut.

- Egg soufflé: Whip egg whites with whisk until fluffy. Stir in yolks. Add Chinese mustard greens, canned crab, garlic, ginger, and raw dairy cheese. Spray pan with coconut oil spray and bake at 375 degrees for 35 minutes until golden brown.

- Sear chicken livers with whole garlic cloves in avocado oil. When almost thoroughly cooked, add oyster mushrooms and yellow zucchini. Burn a little bit. Finish off by tossing in raw sauerkraut, avocado slices, and raw tomatoes. Drizzle with organic ghee and aged balsamic vinegar.

- Tilapia tacos: Warm Julian's Bakery coconut wraps with a little butter in a frying pan. Sear tilapia pieces with curry powder, chipotle sauce, onions, and tomatoes. Add avocados, raw milk cheddar, and organic pastured sour cream.

HCG Phase 4 Friendly Meals (and beyond)

- Gluten free Paleo burger: (stack up neatly in layers) pastured beef patties, egg over easy on top, pastured bacon, raw cheese, Paleo mayo, ketchup from Trinity Hills Farms, lettuce, tomato, and avocado. The bun is made from tapioca starch and brown rice flour.

- In coconut oil, fry pumpkin or butternut squash chunks with salted egg yolk. Serve with steak smothered in raw butter and garlic.

- Fry plantains in coconut oil. Serve with organic sour cream. The resistant starch in plantains is good for energy without sacrificing your desire to stay lean.

- Peruvian Causa: Purée cooked potatoes with saffron, salt, and red pepper paste. Layer potatoes with fresh crab meat, avocado, and pickled onions.

- Sear swordfish in walnut oil. Add kale and spinach to the pan. On the side, halve Vietnamese rice rolls stuffed with raw shredded carrots, basil, and bean sprouts.

- Grill freshwater trout and shrimp with onions and tomatoes. Bake sweet potato fries with a little coconut oil, salt, and pepper.

The places you can go with your innovative ideas and preferred flavor profiles are endless. Let this be a springboard for your personal menu.

PODCASTS
I ENJOY
LISTENING TO

S ince I began my health journey a few years ago I searched for podcasts that would educate me about the truth in nutrition and ask of me new things to think about. If I was intrigued or moved by a show, I would then seek out books by the guest experts in their fields of work. If I liked a show a lot, I would go back and listen to every episode ever made, in chronological order. What a wonderful experience this has been.

The following is my most listened to list of iTunes podcasts:

- HCG Body For Life! (Colin F. Watson)
- HCG Chica (Rayzel Lam)

- Fat Burning Man (Abel James)
- Ben Greenfield Fitness Podcast (Ben Greenfield)
- Low Carb Conversations (Jimmy Moore & Friends)
- The Paleo View (Stacy Toth and Sarah Ballantyne)
- Paleo Lifestyle and Fitness Podcast (Sarah Fragoso and Jason Seib)
- Not Just Paleo (Evan Brand)
- Balanced Bites: Modern Paleo Living (Diane Sanfilippo and Liz Wolfe)
- Ask The Low Carb Experts (Jimmy Moore)
- The Livin' La Vida Low Carb Show (Jimmy Moore)
- Latest in Paleo (Angelo Coppola)
- Revolution Health Radio(Chris Kresser)
- Relentless Roger and the Caveman Doctor (Roger Dickerman & Colin Champ)
- The Paleo Solution Podcast (Robb Wolf)
- Underground Wellness Radio (Sean Croxton)
- The Calorie Myth and Your Smarter Science of Slim (Jonathan Bailor)
- Bulletproof Radio (Dave Asprey)

BIBLIOGRAPHY

Appleton, Nancy and Jacobs, G.N. *Suicide by Sugar: A Startling Look at Our #1National Addiction*. Garden City Park, New York: Square One Publishers, 2009.

Budwig, Dr. Johanna. *The Budwig Cancer and Coronary Heart Disease Prevention Diet: The Revolutionary Diet from Dr. Johanna Budwig, the Woman Who Discovered Omega-3s*. Los Angeles: Freedom Press, 2001.

Budwig, Dr. Johanna. *Flax Oil as a True Aid Against Arthritis, Heart Infraction, Cancer, and Other Diseases*. Denver, Colorado: Apple Tree Publishing Company, 1994.

Burzynski, The Movie. Director, Eric Merola. 2010. DVD.

Cordain, Loren. *The Paleo Diet*. Hoboken, New Jersey: John Wiley and Sons, Inc., 2011.

Daniel, Kaayla T. *The Whole Soy Story: The Dark side of America's Favorite Health Food*. Washington, D. C.: New Trends Publishing, Inc., 2005.

Davis, William. *Wheat Belly*. New York: Rodale, 2011.

Fife, Bruce, M. D. *Coconut Cures: Preventing and Treating Health Problems with Coconut*. Colorado Springs, Colorado: Piccadilly Books, Ltd., 2005.

Graham, Gray, Kesten, Deborah, and Scherwitz, Larry. *Pottenger's Prophecy: How Food Resets Genes for Wellness or Illness*. Amherst, Massachusetts: White River Press, 2011.

Gerson, Charlotte and Walker, Norton, D. P. M. *The Gerson Therapy*. New York, New York: Kensington Books, 2006.

Gundry, Steven R. *Dr. Gundry's Diet Evolution*. New York, New York: Crown Publishers, 2008.

Lustig, Robert H. *Fat Chance: Beating the Odds Against Sugar, Processed Food, Obesity, and Disease*. New York, New York: Plume, 2013.

Lustig, Robert H. *Sugar: The Bitter Truth*. San Francisco: www.uctv.tv, 2009. Filmed Lecture.

Lustig, Robert H. *Fat Chance: Fructose 2.0*. San Francisco: www.uctv.tv, 2013. Filmed Lecture.

Main, Emily. "Boost Your Fat Intake to Save Your Brain." www.rodalenews.com, 2013.

Perlmutter, David. *Grain Brain*. New York, New York: Little, Brown, and Company, 2013.

Sandage, Anji with Bull, Lorena Novak, R. D. *The Everything Coconut Diet Cookbook*. Avon, Massachusetts: Adams Media, 2012.

Simeons, A. T. W. *Pounds and Inches: A New Approach to Obesity*. Rome, Italy: Salvator Mundi International Hospital, 1954.

Simoncini, T. *Cancer is a Fungus: A Revolution in Tumor Therapy*. Rome, Italy: Edizioni, 2007.

Watson, Colin F. *HCG Body for Life: How to Feel Good Naked in 26 Days*. Hermosa Beach, California: Watson Enterprises and Create Space Independent Publishing Platform, 2010.

www.budwigcenter.com

www.budwigvideos.com

www.burzynskiclinic.com

www.burzynskipatientgroup.org

www.cancerisafungus.com

www.curenaturalicancro.com

www.gersoninstitute.org

www.gersonmedia.com

www.theworldshealthiestfoods.org

ABOUT THE AUTHOR

*K*J Landis is her first success story. She lost 50 pounds in 60 days and has kept it off for years. Daily research and coaching has fueled her to help others dive into their own better existences.

KJ Landis is an educator, former model, health and life coach, photographer, and role model. She has inspired many with her holistic approach to health and wellness. Her ability to communicate effectively, compassionately, and with patience has helped build the self esteem and attainment of others' life goals.

She developed a guide based upon her post weight and fat loss journey called Superior Self's Guide to Wellness from Within. It is simple and effective in energy rejuvenation and fat loss. The guide provides a guide to overall wellness and vitality. She teaches wellness workshops all over the San Francisco area based upon the guide.

Currently KJ Landis lives and works in San Francisco with her husband and two children.

CPSIA information can be obtained at www.ICGtesting.com
Printed in the USA
BVOW01s0351151014

370805BV00001B/2/P